AF694065

A PSYCHOANALYTIC STUDY OF LAWRENCE DURRELL'S *THE ALEXANDRIA QUARTET*

A Psychoanalytic Study of Lawrence Durrell's The Alexandria Quartet: *Exile and Return* focuses on the dialogue created by literature and psychoanalysis in an individual's quest to explore existential issues, such as a sense of belonging to a homeland and a recurring sense of the Uncanny (*das unheimliche*). Rony Alfandary explores Durrell's attempt to recreate a sense of belonging to a homeland, which perhaps never existed but can be retraced and reinvented through writing.

This book studies some issues present in Durrell's work:

- the connection between biographical and fictional elements in the study of literature
- the influence of early Freudian theoretical themes upon the writer
- later influences including post-modern and hermeneutic theories

The life and work of Lawrence Durrell can serve as a prototype of a man's quest for meaning, in a world caught in turmoil in the period between and during WW2. The author's psychoanalytic exploration of the work and its relevance to human experience today, shows how the themes Durrell dealt with remain relevant. Alfandary highlights the ways in which his usage of several author narrative styles exemplifies the divergent and often contradictory nature of "Truth", emerging rather as multi-layered, multi-voiced and often torn sense of human subjectivity.

A Psychoanalytic Study of Lawrence Durrell's The Alexandria Quartet: *Exile and Return* demonstrates Durrell's strong influence by psychoanalytic thought and will appeal to both psychoanalytic and literary scholars.

Rony Alfandary, Ph.D., is a clinical social worker, writer and photographer. Rony is a lecturer at Bar-Ilan University in Israel and is in private practice as a psychoanalytic psychotherapist.

A PSYCHOANALYTIC STUDY OF LAWRENCE DURRELL'S *THE ALEXANDRIA QUARTET*

Exile and Return

Rony Alfandary

Routledge
Taylor & Francis Group
LONDON AND NEW YORK

First published 2019
by Routledge
2 Park Square, Milton Park, Abingdon, Oxon OX14 4RN

and by Routledge
711 Third Avenue, New York, NY 10017

Routledge is an imprint of the Taylor & Francis Group, an informa business

© 2019 Rony Alfandary

The right of Rony Alfandary to be identified as author of this work has been asserted by him in accordance with sections 77 and 78 of the Copyright, Designs and Patents Act 1988.

All rights reserved. No part of this book may be reprinted or reproduced or utilised in any form or by any electronic, mechanical, or other means, now known or hereafter invented, including photocopying and recording, or in any information storage or retrieval system, without permission in writing from the publishers.

This book is an expanded translation of a work previously published in Hebrew by Carmel Publishers, Jerusalem as *Exile and Return: A Psychoanalytic Study of Lawrence Durrell's The Alexandria Quartet* (2016).

Translated by the author.

Trademark notice: Product or corporate names may be trademarks or registered trademarks, and are used only for identification and explanation without intent to infringe.

British Library Cataloguing-in-Publication Data
A catalogue record for this book is available from the British Library

Library of Congress Cataloging-in-Publication Data
Names: Alfandary, Rony, author.
Title: A psychoanalytic study of Lawrence Durrell's The Alexandria quartet : exile and return / Rony Alfandary.
Other titles: Galut òve-hitgalut. English
Description: London ; New York, NY : Routledge, 2018. | Includes bibliographical references and index.
Identifiers: LCCN 2018027100 | ISBN 9781138359659 (hardback : alk. paper) | ISBN 9780429782404 (web pdf) | ISBN 9780429782398 (epub) | ISBN 9780429782381 (mobipocket/kindle)
Subjects: LCSH: Durrell, Lawrence. Alexandria quartet. | Psychoanalysis and literature.
Classification: LCC PR6007.U76 A731413 2018 | DDC 823/.912—dc23
LC record available at https://lccn.loc.gov/2018027100

ISBN: 978-1-138-35965-9 (hbk)
ISBN: 978-0-429-43357-3 (ebk)

Typeset in Bembo
by Apex CoVantage, LLC

MIX
Paper from responsible sources
FSC www.fsc.org FSC® C013056

Printed and bound in Great Britain by
TJ International Ltd, Padstow, Cornwall

CONTENTS

Acknowledgements *vi*
Foreword *vii*
A few milestones in the life of Lawrence Durrell *ix*

Introduction: *The Alexandria Quartet* in its contemporary context 1

1 Psychoanalysis, writing and exile 13

2 Whose voice is it anyway? Narratives and structure 36

3 Dreams and dreaming 56

4 The topographic return to the mother-city 74

5 The secret wound 111

6 Epilogue 138

Bibliography *141*
Index *149*

ACKNOWLEDGEMENTS

The book you are about to read was first written in Hebrew and was published in Israel in 2016 by Carmel Publishers as part of the *Psychoanalysis, Hermeneutics and Culture* series, edited by my teacher and Ph.D. tutor Prof. Avi Sagi (Senior Editor) and Dr. Aner Govrin (Associate Editor) of the Program of Hermeneutics and Cultural Studies at Bar-Ilan University. My first thanks goes to them for having an important and supportive role in the previous publication.

The process of translating the Hebrew edition was of course not simple and in fact amounted to a rewriting of the book. I am grateful for the opportunity to rethink some of the ideas in this study. As such, the process of writing can never really come to an end.

I am grateful to Richard Pine for contributing a Foreword and for encouragement and advice while I was preparing this edition. I would also like to thank the members of the International Lawrence Durrell Society, some of whom have shown keen interest in my work in progress. It is a privilege to associate with such a group.

Lastly, I would like to thank my wife and sons whose interest in my work have been constant and provided me with the peace of mind required for such a task. It is with them that I keep finding my home. And very last, my deepest gratitude to my parents, themselves refugees from Second World War Europe, who read the *Quartet* when it came out in England, where they resided at the time.

Rony Alfandary
April 2018

FOREWORD

Studies of the work of Lawrence Durrell, and to a lesser extent of his early associates, Henry Miller and Anaïs Nin, abound in the application of literary theory, most often to the detriment of their work. Durrell has been examined as a postmodernist, an anarchist and a Surrealist, with little light being shed on how we might read his work and scant attention to his own bald statement "I am a Durrealist."

Seldom do we find a sectoral study which prioritises the writer over the theorist. It is therefore all the more valuable that Rony Alfandary has made a study of Durrell's *Alexandria Quartet*, employing his professional acumen as a psychoanalytic psychotherapist to unpack Durrell's writing in terms of the unconscious and the uncanny.

I am particularly interested to see the attention Alfandary pays to Freud's *Uncanny* – that much misunderstood concept of *unheimliche* which, Alfandary shows us, is profoundly present in Durrell's life and art. What he has to say about Durrell's relation to the *unheimliche* Indian background and the constant recurrence of the uncanny in his work is of great value to us all.

So too is what he tells us of the "secret wound" as elaborated by Julia Kristeva. I think it is cognate, but not identical, with what Durrell called the "primal wound" which caused "uprooting despair." It was associated for him with a sense of homelessness and a loss of integration, which gave him, almost from birth, a need to restore wholeness. "The whole course of one's life is simply a search for this lost fragment," he wrote in 1939 and, forty years later, "our life's work is trying to rectify this primal wound."

In *Tunc* Durrell wrote (and I am sure it was autobiographical) of "People deprived of a properly constituted childhood" who suffer from "buried hunger [. . .] aggravated by the sense of emotional impotence." This, and the loss of the Indian "paradise" for which Durrell tried to compensate, indicates to me that Durrell was seeking not only "the jewel in the Lotus" or, in his equally beautiful term, "the primrose in the carnal mind," but appeasement or reconciliation with a world which denied him repose either aesthetically or intellectually.

In *The Black Book*, as early as 1938, he had written "The masked face of myself leans down over my body" and in mid-life, in "The Placebo: an Attic Comedy" Durrell gave us a portrait of a "man in a black hat" revisiting, and being haunted by, the man he once was, and asking "Did he suspect himself of being a poet?" This self-analysis and self-assessment was a continual preoccupation, right up to his death. In *The Dark Labyrinth* he had invented a psychiatrist called Hogarth. When, forty years later, the artist Paul Hogarth published *The Mediterranean Shore: Travels in Lawrence Durrell Country*, Larry gleefully announced to me that nature does imitate art: "At last, I've been analysed by Hogarth!" His juvenile jollity should not blind us to the seriousness with which he regarded the questions of synchronicity, relativity, and duration. Alfandary's study takes us in depth towards an understanding of these factors in Durrell's psychology.

We know that Durrell had read extensively in Freud and Jung even before leaving England at the age of twenty-three. We also know the cardinal moment in 1937, in Paris, when Henry Miller and Anaïs Nin presented him with a copy of Otto Rank's *Art and Artist*. And we are aware of the seminal influence of Georg Groddeck, whose statement "the assertion 'I live' only expresses a small and superficial part of the total experience 'I am lived by the It'" he took thoroughly to heart. It is therefore a special pleasure to encounter an analysis of *The Alexandria Quartet* by someone whose professional life brings him into regular contact with such fellow-analysts and who is thereby enabled to look at Durrell's work in the same spirit as he himself might have wished to do so. Alfandary's couch is where Durrell lies (in both senses of the word).

It is regrettably true, as Rony Alfandary points out, that Durrell's work does not enjoy the same level of popularity as it did during his lifetime, and that even in the wake of *The Alexandria Quartet*, when readers and critics hoped for "more of the same," the novels which followed – *Tunc*, *Nunquam* and *The Avignon Quintet* – were not as well received as his masterpiece, the *Quartet*. But, with his centenary in 2012, marked not only by major conferences in London and Corfu but also by a new printing of the *Quartet* (with an Introduction by Jan Morris), an edition of the previously unpublished *Judith* and a CD from the British Library/BBC of his own readings and interviews, attention to Durrell's thought, as well as his work, will begin to intensify. This book contributes significantly to that interest.

Rony Alfandary's book earns its place in the long history of significant *Quartet* studies, from Alan Warren Friedman's *Art for Love's Sake* (1970) and Corinne Alexandre-Garner's *Etude sur l'amour, la femme et l'ecriture* (1985) to Ravindran Nambiar's *Indian Metaphysics in Lawrence Durrell's Novels* (2014). If he can persuade himself to look at *Tunc/Nunquam* and *The Avignon Quintet* in a later study I hope Rony Alfandary will continue the Ariadne's thread of exploration both towards, and back from, the other minotaurs lurking in Durrell's labyrinth.

Richard Pine
Durrell Library of Corfu

A FEW MILESTONES IN THE LIFE OF LAWRENCE DURRELL[1]

27 February, 1912	Born in Jalandhar, India.
1915	Margery (sister) is born but dies after several months.
1917	Leslie (brother) is born.
1919	Margaret (sister) is born.
1921	Sent to a Jesuit boarding school, St. Joseph's, in Darjeeling, India.
1923	Leaves India, accompanied by his parents and brother and sister. Parents and sister return to India while he begins school.
1924	Louisa (mother) visits England and returns to India with Leslie. Lawrence enrols in St. Olave's and St. Xavier's Grammar School in Southwark, London.
1925	Gerald (brother) is born. The Durrells visit Lawrence in England.
1926	Lawrence Samuel (father) visits England and buys a house in Dulwich. Lawrence is enrolled in St. Edmund's boarding school in Canterbury.
1928	Lawrence Samuel dies in India, age 43. Louisa and the children leave India and settle in Dulwich.
1929	Lawrence leaves Canterbury, as widowed Louisa cannot afford to keep him there. She sells house in Dulwich and moves to rented accommodation. Lawrence begins to spend more time in London on his own.
1931	Moves to London and publishes his first collection of poetry.
1932	Meets Nancy Isobel Myers.

1935	Marries his first wife Nancy in London. Moves to Corfu with Nancy. Persuades his mother (who is in bad health) to move with him. His brothers and sister join the group. After a short while, Lawrence and Nancy find their own house on the island. Publishes first novel, *Pied Piper of Lovers.*
1937	Publishes his second novel, *Panic Spring.* Visits Paris with Nancy. Meets Henry Miller for the first time.
1938	Returns to Corfu. Publication of *The Black Book* by Obelisk Press in Paris.
1939	Lawrence and Nancy move to Athens.
1940	Birth of first daughter, Penelope Berengaria Durrell in Athens.
1941	Moves to Cairo, Egypt. Works as junior press officer as well as co-founding a poetry journal *Personal Landscape.*
1942	First Issue of *Personal Landscape,* including his poetry. Moves to Alexandria. Nancy leaves him and takes their daughter to Palestine.
1943	Meets Yvette (Eve) Cohen. Works on *Prospero's Cell,* a book about his time in Cyprus.
1944	*Personal Lanscape* has its 7th issue. Corresponds with Henry Miller about his intention to write about Alexandria.
1945	Moves to Rhodes to work as director of public relations for the Overseas Information Service. Works on *The Dark Labyrinth.*
1947	Marries second wife, Eve Cohen, after divorcing first wife, Nancy.
1948	Moves to Argentina to lecture at the University of Cordoba.
1949	Moves to Yugoslavia where he works as press attache.
1951	Birth of second daughter, Sappho Jane.
1953	Moves to Cyprus, where he teaches in Nicosia.
1954	Separates from Eve, his second wife.
1955	Meets Claude-Marie Vincendon. They move in together in Cyprus.
1957	Moves to the south of France with Claude. Eve divorces him.
1957–1959	Writes and publishes *The Alexandria Quartet (Justine, Balthazar, Mountolive, Clea).*
1961	Marries third wife, Claude.
1964	Louisa Durrell (mother) dies in England.
1966	Durrell and Claude buy the house in Sommières where he spends the rest of his life.
1967	Claude dies on January 1st, at the age of 42, having been diagnosed with cancer after several months of ill health. Durrell is devastated.

1968–1970	Publishes *Tunc* and *Nunquam*.
1973	Marries his fourth wife, Ghislaine de Boysson. They divorce in 1977.
1974–1985	Publishes *The Avignon Quintet*.
1985	Daughter Sappho takes her own life.
7 November 1990	During the last years of his life lives with Françoise Kestsman. Dies and is cremated; his ashes are buried in Sommières near the grave of Claude.

Note

1 For a comprehensive and updated chronology of Durrell's life, the best source is the one kept online in the Durrell Library of Corfu and compiled by Brewster Chamberlin. www.durrelllibrarycorfu.org.

INTRODUCTION

The Alexandria Quartet in its contemporary context

"You are writing a book about Lawrence Durrell? Really? Does anyone know who he was? Does anyone remember him?" Such were the customary responses to the writing of this book.

More so, as the first edition of the book was written in Hebrew and was circulated only in Israel, the disbelief was even greater.[1] It is hard to find copies of his books in most bookshops in England, which some would say could be regarded as his *cultural homeland*.[2] This state of affairs is perhaps the lot of most writers, especially in the period immediately following their death and therefore perhaps does not even merit mention. Nevertheless, the mere mention of the term *homeland* in reference to the origins of Lawrence George Durrell (1912–1990) is a complex issue which I will discuss in subsequent chapters. Suffice to say at this point that Durrell, whose birthplace was India, where he was born to colonial Anglo-Indian parents, felt ill at ease in England and continued to have a very divided and ambivalent relation towards a-place-he-could-call-home. At best, one could say that Durrell felt really at home in the contradictory sense implied by the German word *das unheimliche*. This term, translated as *the Uncanny*, became central in Western culture since it was interpreted by Sigmund Freud (1856–1939) and denotes both homeliness and its opposite, strangeness.[3] As Freud writes in his 1919 essay: "*Heimlich* is a word the meaning of which develops in the direction of ambivalence, until it finally coincides with its opposite, *unheimliche. Unheimliche* is in some way or other a sub-species of *Heimlich*. Let us bear this discovery in mind, though we cannot yet rightly understand it."[4] Based upon his interpretation of a short story by the Prussian author E.T.A. Hoffman (1776–1822), Freud concluded that we tend to experience the *unheimliche* sensation when we are not sure whether what we see is alive or dead, real or artificial. He suggested that that feeling originates from an early stage in the development of the infant when he invents a duplicate sense of himself in order to deal with terrifying events that he cannot integrate or understand with his budding rational faculties. The duplicate sense of self, later finding an echo in the term *Doppelgänger*, loses its functionality as we mature, but leaves its trace in the unconscious layers of our mind. Later in life, when we encounter complexities and ambivalences in our relation to, and perception of, the world around us, we are linked, according to Freud, to that relic in our minds and experience the *unheimliche* sensation. The notions of the *unheimliche*, *belonging* and *home* are central to my study and will be discussed in depth in later chapters.

In this brief introduction, I will outline some of the critical and cultural contexts that place Durrell within a particular field among his contemporaries. I shall deal with the question of the apparent, and hopefully temporary, demise of his popularity in the fifth and final chapter of the book.

Durrell's main project in his writing was the constitution of his inner world as a place he could call his home. His personal circumstances made him perceive himself as a solitary being looking out on the world from his aloof and distant position. Such an experience of solitude made him emphasise the endeavours of the individual for self-fulfilment when his environment was experienced as alien and often inferior. He drew inspiration from his surrounding, but did not always fully acknowledge its immense value in constituting his identity as a writer.

Durrell's star first appeared in the sky of Western culture during the late 1950s, with the publication of the *Quartet*, which won him two Nobel nominations in the 1960s, albeit never actually securing the prize. Nowadays, he is mostly known as the brother of zoologist Gerald Durrell (1925–1995), author of the best-selling *My Family and Other Animals*, among other works.[5] But Durrell and his oeuvre nevertheless remain relevant to this day. His life and work epitomise the quest for meaning of the modern man in the Western world in the latter half of the twentieth century.

It may come as a surprise to the English reader that Durrell was known in Israel in the 1960s.[6] He wrote the screenplay for *Judith*, the first international motion picture shot in Israel with American funding, starring Sophia Loren (born 1934) and Peter Finch (1916–1977). He stayed in Israel in 1962 during some of the shooting and even met the legendary Israeli Prime Minister of that time, David Ben-Gurion (1886–1973). The film follows the tale of a young woman, played by Loren, who arrives in Palestine as an illegal immigrant having survived the horrors of the Holocaust in 1944. The location of the production and the filming set near Kibbutz Shamir were the focus of much attention. It was rescreened in 2014 as part of the Haifa International Film Festival.

Durrell's connection with Jewish people went beyond that. Two of his four wives were Jewish. Moreover, the plot of *The Alexandria Quartet*, as will be shown later, also has as its focus the tale of Justine, an Egyptian-Jewish woman from an Alexandrian family, whose character is partly based on that of Eve (Yvette) Cohen (1918–2004), Durrell's second wife. A significant narrative focal point in the novel, as I will explore in detail in chapters four and five, deals with the subject of arms smuggling from Egypt to Palestine by the Jewish underground before the state of Israel came into existence in 1948.

Perhaps Durrell's romantic enchantment with the Jewish homeland was no coincidence, as was his later interest and involvement in the local politics in several of the places he had found himself in. He himself was a man who could not easily call anywhere *home* nor belong clearly to *a homeland*. Born in India to parents of British origins, he was sent to a prestigious boarding school in England as a youth, but hated it with passion.[7] He was a citizen of the world and a man of no nationality.[8] The circumstances of his life and work meant that he travelled from one country to another, searching for a place he could call his home. For Durrell, writing *The Alexandria Quartet* meant working through his complex sense of affiliation with his homeland – be it actual or imaginary.

Durrell was also deeply preoccupied by his search for truth. As he put it through the voice of one of the minor protagonists in the book, the journalist John Keats, truth was not a specific tool one could wield, nor did it promise to be revealed easily or even be very reliable. But he did firmly believe that through the use of words one can achieve what was his ultimate goal in life – to grow-up and mature into a creative truthful human being.[9] Therefore, as I will argue in the first chapter of the book, it should be no surprise that his work relied on psychoanalytical insights offered by several thinkers who had inspired him. Durrell formed a curious relationship with psychoanalytic theory, and allowed its influence to be part of his life. In later chapters I will discuss his ambivalent relationship with his father, who sent him away to a boarding school when he was eleven and died himself five years later, thus creating a tangled knot in his consciousness which I will refer to as *the secret wound*. It is no surprise therefore that he actually felt closest to those psychoanalysts who had a complex relationship with their father, or their father figure (Freud), as was the case with Otto Rank (1884–1939), Carl Jung (1875–1961) and Georg Groddeck (1866–1934).

The psychoanalytic insights employed in this book are not meant to place Durrell on the couch. The object of this book is to trace his personal quest for meaning and sense in life while being guided with psychoanalytic ideas that he himself was aware of and used in his own writing. As I will argue in later chapters, the circumstances of his existence create a special psychic urge for such a quest. It is through his writing that he had tried to respond to that inner quest. Reading the *Quartet* is akin to listening to his quest, in a way which is not entirely dissimilar to the kind of listening that is required in therapy. Being a psychotherapist myself, I read the *Quartet* and search for Durrell's voice in it, as well as my own. Reading the *Quartet* is therefore not just a reflection and testimony of the maturational process Durrell has gone through, but also creates such a platform for the informed and willing reader.

Cultural contexts

The following pages will trace some of the cultural contexts that influence and guide Durrell's work, and the circumstances surrounding its publication and reception in the light of Harold Bloom's (born 1930) seminal work on *poetic influence*.[10] Bloom claimed that an author can never be read in isolation and that each author can be read only through reading other authors. Using *the family* as a metaphor, Bloom claims that reading a poet involves meeting and accepting all his relatives as well, in the same way that we cannot allow a new member into our family circle without his own family and family history too. The Israeli scholar Avidav Lipskar claims that examining the status and quality of literary work is not aimed towards providing an explanation.[11] It is not enough to try to explain what the work is about, nor is it sufficient to delve into an analysis of the character and life circumstances of the author in order to get a good appreciation of the text. The questions *why was the work written as such?* or *what made the author write such a text?* create a critical vacuum which distances the reader from appreciating and living the possibilities inherent within the text. A text need not be understood so much as be absorbed and make sense to the reader in the sense that it makes an existential difference to their life.[12] Lipskar suggests an examination of the work within its cultural ecological field to allow a phenomenological study of its merits.[13]

Once *The Alexandria Quartet* was published in the late 1950s, Durrell became a renowned figure in literary circles the world over. The work was translated into many languages and enjoyed considerable commercial success. Critically too, the *Quartet* attracted considerable attention, and Durrell was cited alongside the likes of Marcel Proust (1871–1922) and James Joyce (1882–1941), and enjoyed the attention and appreciation of T.S. Eliot (1888–1965), chief editor of the prestigious publishing house Faber & Faber, who published Durrell's books. Eliot had already paid favourable critical attention to Durrell when he wrote after the publication of *The Black Book* in 1938:

> Lawrence Durrell's *The Black Book* is the first piece of work by a new English writer to give me any hope for the future of prose fiction. If he has been influenced by any writers of my generation and the influences digested, he has produced something different. One test of the book's qualities for me, is the way in which reminiscences of it keep turning up in my mind. . . . *The Black Book* is not a scrap-book, but a carefully executed whole. There is nothing of the second-hand literary about the material. What is most unusual is the structure the author has made of it.[14]

The *Quartet* and the works that followed found their way into the curriculums of literature courses in different universities worldwide. Monographs were dedicated to different aspects of Durrell's work. As his close friend Anaïs Nin (1903–1977) wrote:

> There was a Durrell epidemic. As he announced there were more books to come, I felt he was going to write the book of our century, as Proust did in his time. I was consoled to think that civilized, developed, full-blown literature was at last recognized in America: that Puritanism had lost its battle for the short, Anglo-Saxon words as against the Latinized roots. That wealth of vocabulary, wealth of images and all the excesses of a Byzantine court had become part of our daily reading.[15]

The Alexandria Quartet was perceived to epitomise the modernist *zeitgeist* of 1960s Europe and North America, providing a source of inspiration for many writers and artists. Durrell's unique outlook on *modern love*, with his emphasis on unfettered expressions of sexuality as a leitmotif of the freedom of the individual, can be seen in the context of the liberal trends of the 1960s.[16] Darley, the main protagonist of the *Quartet*, whose perspective occupies most of the narrative, recognises love as the ultimate and absolute entity, an entity worth sacrificing all for. In his view, the individual should be prepared to risk all that he has, including his position in society, for the sake of the fulfilment of love.[17]

The position that Lawrence Durrell held in society was of a white man born in the Orient, who spent the better part of his life in a quest for an actual or imaginary affiliation in an alienated modern world, and became an inspirational figure among his contemporaries.[18] His lifelong search for self-fulfilment was very much in harmony with the humanistic tendencies of the time. His life and writing carve out a figure of an Anglo-Saxon artist on a quest for his true identity in remote geographical regions, representing perhaps his yearning to reach deep into the recess of his psyche to recapture a primeval experience that may restore the lost meaning to his life.[19]

The *Quartet* is replete with statements made by Darley, and others, of existential despair. That despair is described as the current state of affairs of people in his circumstances, a sense of despair that could create a bonding with other human beings in a similar situation. These others were characters in the novel, but also refer to the readers of the *Quartet* at that time, reflecting the sense of despair in post–Second World War Europe. Humanity has taken a blow, and it is only through the individual search for meaning and salvation, perhaps through love, that redemption was possible.[20]

Literary beginnings

In 1935, after he had moved to Corfu, he was given a copy of Henry Miller's (1891–1980) first published novel *Tropic of Cancer*.[21] Reading Miller's book and having left England, where his father had sent him to acquire "proper" education and which he hated, calling it *Pudding Island*, mark one of the key moments in his life.[22] This instance demonstrates the impact that reading had upon the course of his life. Miller's book opened a door for him into a world he had hitherto only experienced from afar. The experience of reading and meeting Miller gave him the inner licence to write in ways he could only dream until then. Miller was the inspiration Durrell had required in order to come out of his shell as an author, as he did later with the publication of *The Black Book* in 1938. As he wrote to Miller in his first letter to him in 1935:

> Strikes me as being the only really man-size piece of work which this century can really boast of. It's a howling triumph from the word go; and not only is it a literary and artistic smack on the bell for everyone, but it really gets down on paper the blood and bowels of our time. I have never read anything like it. I did not imagine anything like it could be written; and yet, curiously,

> reading it I seemed to recognise it as something which I knew we're all ready for [. . .] I salute *Tropic* as the copy-book for my generation.[23]

Both *Tropic of Cancer* and *The Black Book* received their share of censorship, due to the allegedly obscene contents of their books, with their explicit sexual allusions. It was only twenty years later that their full distribution was allowed in the US and Britain. The *Quartet*, which was published twenty years after *The Black Book*, also contained explicit sexual accounts, as will be discussed in chapter four. The explicit sexual contents earned it immediate attention, marking it as one of the hallmarks of the permissive, liberal mood that characterised the 1960s, so different in nature to that which prevailed when Durrell and Miller began to write. The different official receptions of *The Black Book* and The *Quartet* show perhaps the change in the way sexuality was treated in the public eye. Durrell's letters from the 1930s show that he was revelling in the fact that the establishment viewed his works as a challenge to the present social order on account of the explicit mention of sexuality. He enjoyed his image as an anti-establishment author.

Durrell and his first wife, Nancy Myers (1912–1983), spent a few months during 1937–1938 in Paris in the company of Miller, Anaïs Nin and the Austrian writer Alfred Perlès (1897–1990). Durrell was then exposed to bohemian, creative life that changed him, providing him with new channels of thought that were to guide him from then on. Up until then, Durrell had been mostly inspired by the Romantic and Elizabethan English literature tradition. His exposure to the ideas and activities of the Surrealist movement in Paris and the introduction to international artists like writer Alfred Perlès (1897–1990), photographer Man Ray (1890–1976), poet and writer André Breton (1896–1966), photographer Brassaï (1899–1984), art historian and critic Herbert Read (1893–1968) and poet David Gascoyne (1916–2001) provided an inspiration to his future work.[24] Durrell became actively involved in editing and bringing to print literary projects that offered a platform for avant-garde, at times pornographic, materials that defied the social norms of his period.[25] Durrell's efforts enjoyed the attention of writers like George Orwell (1903–1950) and his mentor T.S. Eliot. The commercial failure of these publications and the deluge of puritan response in their wake only forged his resolve to pursue writing, driven by the notion that he was marching in the forefront of a cultural movement that was about to change the face of the world.[26]

Politics and style

The contact with the political base of the Surrealist movement, be it the anarchist or the Marxist faction, eventually drove him away from it. His disenchantment with those clear political ideas informed the course of his involvement outside his own room. He resolved to make writing his sole arena, the place where he could make a difference. He espoused aesthetic and philosophic ideas that held the creative process as the only process that allowed modern man full expression. He viewed external change in the life of the individual as less relevant to his personal growth and development as an artist. As he wrote to Miller in 1936: "This manifesto would be a lot clearer if these brave young revolutionaries started by defining what they mean by art. . . . [P]olitics are not going to be confused with art. I'm tired of political people. They have confused the inner struggle with the outer one."[27] It was not just the political aspect of Surrealism that put Durrell off in those days. He remained averse to all political movements in later years as he saw them as opposing artistic endeavour. In the *Quartet*, twenty years later, he referred to Marxism with his not unusual tongue-in-cheek humour verging on racism through the lips of Pursewarden, one of the protagonists and narrative voices of the *Quartet*, saying its appearance was proof of the Jews and the Irish taking revenge on society.[28]

This polarisation of art versus politics followed Durrell throughout his life. He adopted a conservative, individualistic position that invested the individual and his self-fulfilment with the uttermost value. He coined the term *the Heraldic Universe*, which I will explore in chapter four, to justify his isolationist position. It is his view of himself as a universe unto himself which explains such remarks as he made in one of his letters to Miller:

> You say in big strident tones: I AM A MAN. THAT IS ENOUGH. Because you know that an artist can hardly taste his food – he is so weak with virtue. If it were possible you would like to go on saying I AM A MAN ad lib in order to hide the more terrible stage whisper I AM AN ARTIST and from there to the ultimate blinding conclusion IAMGOD!!! It is this role which confuses you by its limitless scope. And it is this area of the soul that germ of the final thunderclap is breeding.[29]

The isolationist position Durrell adopted, whereby he saw himself as belonging to no particular intellectual circle, could perhaps also be attributed to the fact he had never undergone formal academic training. Still, this did not mean he remained ignorant to the wealth of literature and culture around him.[30] On the contrary, he made up for this apparent lack with voracious and diverse reading. His library now scattered among several universities and research centres around the world, comprised thousands of volumes in several languages. Scholars can observe his handwritten notes, mostly written in the margins, in most of these books. He read and employed his reading in his own writing. Durrell drew his inspiration from whatever he read – Ancient Greek and Latin literature, Elizabethan poets and playwrights, Surrealists, psychoanalytical theoreticians, modern literature and poetry and Buddhist and Taoist scriptures, to cite but a few.[31] As Durrell himself confessed, almost everything that he read found its way into his work one way or the other.[32] In his writing he strove to circulate fresh air into what he found to be the stultifying contemporary approach to the issues of modern life, creativity and sexuality. His views of sexuality, which were inspired by psychoanalysis, for example, stood up against the conservative, censorial attitude that he and his fellow poets, like John Gawsworth (1912–1970), identified as the oppressive experience which he would refer to as *the English death*.[33] His views on the fate of English poetry under the oppressive weight of *Pudding Island* were expressed succinctly by Darley in the *Quartet*, as he walks with his lover, the painter Clea, amongst some ruins where he imagines he is seeing rats, he prays to God to spare him their wrath despite the fact that he is an English poet.[34]

His literary style was described as Baroque, drawing on different styles and influences, from Elizabethan poetry, through metaphysical poetry, to the work of D.H. Lawrence (1885–1930).[35] George Steiner (born 1929) identified Durrell's literary style as rich and musical, unlike the prevalent literary style of the period, which was lean and purposefully poor of vocabulary, like the prose Ernest Hemingway (1899–1961) wrote:

> Nothing is ever explained . . . language falls upon the reader's senses like brocade . . . the style is mosaic. Each word is set in its precise and luminous place . . . no one else writing in English today has quite the same commitment to the light and music of language.[36]

Durrell wrote in a rich and luscious style so as to proclaim himself a literary universe unto himself.

His aloof position, seemingly unfettered by any literary tradition, is nevertheless saturated with the many influences that he absorbed through his reading. His writing can be romantic, postmodernist or journalistic, often determined by what he was writing. Whether he was writing poetry,[37] prose, drama,[38] light humorous pieces[39] or *foreign residence* literature,[40] he always remained Lawrence Durrell. His writing, having reached its peak in the *Quartet*, conforms to no particular literary formula, therefore generating a rich matrix of consciousness that often feels challenging and fragmentary, reflecting his troubled and rich mind.[41]

Influence

When trying to understand what happened when Durrell began to lose critical acclaim, there are several points to consider. Michael Begnal argues that it is hard, and even impossible, to characterise Durrell's extraordinarily diverse oeuvre in a way that would facilitate, for example, a reissue of his work. [42] It is this point that T.S. Eliot had in mind during the 1940s when he implored Durrell to make the choice of pursuing a career as either a novelist or a poet.[43] Durrell did not listen to his advice or similar advice from Miller, who urged him to focus on his own work rather than investing too much effort in publishing selected works by Miller. Charles Sligh argues too that the overall Durrell oeuvre is not typical of the conventional oeuvre, where one can trace a linear progression and a gradual thematic development.[44] Such a course of development in the work of a writer allows a certain expectation to emerge. Durrell does not fit into that cubicle. This, according to Sligh, is also where his greatness lies. The fact that he can comfortably write in different genres allows the reader to delve into the texts themselves, with no overall dominant, encapsulating style. None of the texts written by Durrell prepares the reader for the text that would follow. Such deliberate lack of uniformity in the eclectic Durrell oeuvre places him within the postmodern field and can be seen to place obstacles for some readers, who might feel more comfortable with more uniformity and continuity in the author's corpus. As Richard Pine (born 1949) writes, there are at least three *Lawrence Durrells* who carry an authentic voice as authors. Any comparison between the three, any effort to apply the same critical tools on his overall corpus, will inevitably produce a superficial yield.[45] A different view is taken by James M. Clawson in a recent study of Durrell's novels. By studying Durrell's twelve major novels, Clawson claims that several distinctive and recurring themes can be identified in his work, therefore allowing Durrell's work to be considered as an opus and a single ongoing project.[46]

Durrell's huge critical and commercial popularity in the 1960s dwindled with his later publications. Terry Eagleton (born 1943) criticised Durrell rather acidly using the very same terms that had earned him his reputation in the first place.[47] Eagleton found Durrell's style facile and exotic, out of touch with any real human experience. He described Durrell himself as a brattish author who had spent a lifetime on a protracted holiday. Eagleton argued that the time Durrell spent in different countries could not be seen as exile, but rather as an ongoing quest for a nice sunny place to live in. He believed that the comparison once drawn with the writing of Vladimir Nabokov (1899–1977) and Joyce was misleading, as those writers had grown within a cultural tradition and tried to set themselves apart from it, while Durrell had made no real effort to reckon with his native imperialistic culture. Eagleton employed the term *supreme trickster* to describe Durrell's entire oeuvre as literary embellishments and antics.

A more balanced view, though still critical, was expressed by Martin Green, who was unconvinced of the literary merit of Durrell's oeuvre, claiming that it was only the *Quartet* and his poetry and travel literature that held their ground in perspective.[48] Green was also derisive of the myth of Durrell as the expatriate author, fostered by Durrell himself with the help of Henry Miller and others, and argued that Durrell's quest had been a quest for a convenient life, unencumbered by real challenges.

I find both criticisms to be rather sensational in nature. Their timing coincided with a tidal disapproval of Durrell and his work in the years that followed the release of excerpts from the diary of his second daughter, Sappho Durrell (1951–1985).[49] The journalist Barbara Robson made allegations, based upon her interpretation of those diaries, published posthumously after Sappho's suicide in 1991, that Durrell had had a sexual relationship with her, following the death of his third wife.[50] As Sappho and Durrell were already dead by then, those allegations could not be addressed by the people involved and left an indelible stain on Durrell's reputation and integrity. As will be described in the fifth chapter, Durrell may indeed have been a very difficult father to live with after the death of his beloved wife. The emotional atmosphere in the Sommières house in the south of France was not easy. A close reading of Sappho's diaries does testify to the emotional hardship she endured and to her grave mental condition, but they do not explicitly or even implicitly state that Lawrence Durrell mistreated her sexually.

In summary, despite the decline in popularity, Lawrence Durrell still leaves his mark and can be traced in the work of quite a few other writers, like Kathy Acker (1944–1997), Anthony Burgess (1917–1993), Peter Porter (1929–2010), Julio Cortázar (1914–1984), André Brink (1935–2015), Kazuo Ishiguro (born 1954), M. G. Vassanji (born 1950), Michael Ondaatje (born 1943), and Thomas Pynchon (born 1937). Durrell's oeuvre, as well as Miller's, can also be seen in relation, perhaps in contrast with the 1960s British Angry Young Men. The contempt of this movement towards any literary genre preoccupied mainly with form and content and less so with social realism, often resulted in poor literature. Durrell's treatment of sexuality in the 1950s and 1960s secures him a place of honour in the history of English literature. Inspired by D. H. Lawrence (1885–1930), Durrell proved that sexual experiences could be written about without resorting to the blunt, obscene language employed by his friend Henry Miller. Durrell wrote about sex and sexuality as he wrote about nature, with a sensual, lively and inspiring language.

Today, more than a century after his birth, the work of Lawrence Durrell stands at a crossroads.[51] It does not enjoy the commercial success and critical favour of the 1960s and 1970s, but academic interest in it persists. In the 1980s, The International Lawrence Durrell Society (ILDS) was founded, and holds bi-yearly international conferences, publishes the *Deus Loci* journal and supports new monographs on Durrell's work.[52] The same decade saw a writing school and library set-up by Richard Pine in Corfu, since it had been Durrell's home, where workshops and conferences are held, dedicated to his works and the works of fellow authors.[53] Far from being forgotten, Durrell's overall literary oeuvre, like that of many other authors past their prime, awaits its revival. New editions of his books are available, translated into many languages (the *Quartet* has recently been translated into Serbian). His manuscripts are still unearthed and edited for print. Two recent examples are the publication of the novel rendition of *Judith*, which Durrell wrote in 1968 based on his 1962 Hollywood script for the film shot in Israel, and *The Placebo*, the draft for Durrell's later novels *Tunc* and *Nunquam*, which Richard Pine and David Roessel edited in 2018. The TV series, *The Durrells* will soon go into its fourth season and though it is no substitute for a critical study it does attest to the interest Durrell's work may excite.

The first chapter of the book seeks to clarify the theoretical concepts that will form the basis for the interpretation of *The Alexandria Quartet*. The second chapter explores the different narrative voices of the *Quartet* in the light of Freud's topographical models of the mind. The third chapter explores the way dreams and the language of dreams permeated the *Quartet* and informed its plot and structure. The fourth chapter looks at the city of Alexandria with its symbolic status as a liminal stage in Durrell's development towards returning to his lost primeval homeland. The fifth and final chapter explores the life of Durrell through the binary of biographical and fictional elements strewn throughout his writing. I invite the reader to a journey into the labyrinthine mind of Lawrence Durrell as it showed itself in the writing of *The Alexandria Quartet*. My book has been written based on the assumption that contemporary readers are not acquainted with the work.[54] I therefore provide ample details as to its contents, but still, I strongly recommend reading the *Quartet* itself alongside.

Notes

1 The Hebrew edition was well-received and merited favourable mention in the literary press. For further details see Ziffer, Benny, 2017, "Why was I so happy to see Alfandary's Exile and Return" (Hebrew), in *Haaretz*, January 11th. https://www.haaretz.co.il/literature/study/1.3230353.

2 This study is based upon reading the *Quartet* in its four individual volume edition. Nowadays, these separate volumes can only be found in second-hand bookshops. The current edition of

the *Quartet* can only be bought as a single volume. There are some differences between the different editions which nevertheless do not adversely affect the insights of this study.

3 Throughout the book I use the original German term rather then its English translation as I find that the original word conveys better the deeper sense of this complex term. Without getting involved in an unwarranted etymological discussion, I shall just point out that the original term is composed of the word Heimat which translated as homeland or home which is central to the way Freud used the term. This depth of meaning is lacking in the English translation.

4 Freud, Sigmund, 1919, "The Uncanny", in J. Strachey, ed., *The Standard Edition of the Complete Psychological Works of Sigmund Freud*, trans. J. Strachey, Vol. XVII, London: Hogarth Press, p. 226.

5 In this book, Gerald Durrell described in a light-hearted way the years that the family spent on the Greek Island of Corfu. Lawrence himself features of course in this account, which had recently been televised for the UK commercial channel ITV. For the full account, read Durrell, Gerald, 2016 (1956), *My Family and Other Animals*, London: Macmillan Collector's Library. For a survey of that period, read Haag, Michael, 2017, *The Durrells of Corfu*, London: Profile Books.

6 The *Quartet* is yet to be fully translated into Hebrew. *Justine* was first translated and published in the early 1960s as a single volume. Twenty years later a different translation of *Justine* and *Balthazar* were published.

7 The exact details of Durrell's ancestral roots are a matter of debate. Durrell himself had claimed to have Irish roots but later contradicted himself. He was most likely of English ancestry, as Michael Haag demonstrated in his internet blog – Haag Michael, 2012a, *Lawrence Durrell: In an Irish Fairy's Armpit*, http://michaelhaag.blogspot.com/2012/11/lawrence-durrell-in-irish-fairys-armpit.html

8 He was in fact without a legal national affiliation for many years until he was granted French citizenship after he had been residing in France since the 1960s.

9 Durrell, Lawrence, 1960, *Clea*, London: Faber & Faber, p. 184.

10 Bloom, Harold, 1997, *The Anxiety of Influence*, New York and Oxford: Oxford University Press.

11 Lipskar, Avidav, 2009, "Barriers: Liminal Thresholds in A. B. Yehoshua's Ethical Geography", *Democratic Culture*, 11:169–181.

12 Merav Roth wrote a fascinating study in Hebrew, *Reading the Reader*, published in 2017, where she offers Kleinian-inspired analysis of the way reading facilitates within the reader psychological processes. Her book is due to be published by Routledge later this year.

13 For further reading concerning the literary traditions that Durrell was a part of, read Richard Pine's *Lawrence Durrell: The Mindscape*, published by the Durrell School of Corfu in 2005 (2nd Edition).

14 MacNiven, Ian S., 1998, *Lawrence Durrell: A Biography*, London: Faber & Faber, p. 172.

15 Nin, Anäis, 1967, *The Journals of Anäis Nin, Vol. Six 1955–1966*, London: Quartet Books, p. 103.

16 Bauman, Zygmunt, 2003, *Liquid Love*, Cambridge: Polity Press.

17 Durrell, Lawrence, 1957a, *Justine*, London: Faber & Faber, p. 105.

18 Alexandre-Garner, Corinne, 1997, "The Enigma of the Quartet", in Robert Ilbert, ed., *Alexandria 1960–1980: The Brief Life of a Cosmopolitan Community*, Alexandria: Harpocrete Publishing, pp. 162–167.

19 Kaplan, Caren, 1996, *Questions of Travel, Postmodern Discourses of Displacement*, Durham: Duke University Press, pp. 125–129.

20 Durrell, Lawrence, 1957a, *Justine*, London: Faber & Faber, pp. 22–23.

21 Cleyet, George, 1980, "The Villa Seurat Circle: Creative Nexus", *Deus Loci*, 4:4–6.

22 Durrell had in fact already moved away from London to Corfu at that time, where he resided with his first wife. For more detailed chronological description of that time, refer to Hodgkin, Joanna, 2013, *Amateurs in Eden: The Story of a Bohemian Marriage: Nancy and Lawrence Durrell*, London: Virago.

23 MacNiven, Ian S., 1988, ed. *The Durrell-Miller Letters, 1935–1980*, London: Faber & Faber, p. 2.
24 Brassaï, 1995, *Henry Miller: The Paris Years*, New York: Arcade Publishing, pp. 199–205; Perlès, Alfred, 1961, *My Friend Lawrence Durrell*, Northwood: Scorpion Press, p. 10.
25 The story of the way those publications came into existence, changed hands and direction and finally came to a sorry end is a fascinating and telling one but again not within the scope of this book. For more details about the 'Booster/Delta' epoch and the way the 'Villa Seurat' group lived, one can refer to MacNiven's (1998) account, pp. 166–231.
26 Mackworth, Cecily, 1987, "Montparnasse and 18 Villa Seurat", *Twentieth Century Literature: A Scholarly and Critical Journal*, 33:274–279.
27 MacNiven, Ian S., 1988, ed. *The Durrell-Miller Letters, 1935–1980*, London: Faber & Faber, pp. 17–18.
28 Durrell, Lawrence, 1958b, *Mountolive*, London: Faber & Faber, p. 64.
29 Wickes, George, 1963, *Lawrence Durrell & Henry Miller: A Private Correspondence: Letters of Lawrence Durrell and Henry Miller 1935–1959*, London: E. P. Dutton & Co., Inc., p. 53. The words 'IAMGOD' appear so in the original.
30 Kaczvinksy, Donald, 1993, "Classical and Medieval Sources for Lawrence Durrell", *Notes on Contemporary Literature*, 23:11–12.
31 Dawson, Carl, 1970, "From Einstein to Keats", *Far Eastern Forum*, 1:109–127.
32 Pine, Richard, 2005, *Lawrence Durrell: The Mindscape*, Corfu: Durrell School of Corfu; Ingersoll, Earl G., 1998, *Lawrence Durrell: Conversations*, London: Associated University Press, pp. 105–106.
33 Gawsworth, John, 1969, "My Friend Lawrence Durrell", *Book Collecting & Library Monthly*, 15:80–81
34 Durrell, Lawrence, 1960, *Clea*, London: Faber & Faber, p. 147.
35 Ingalls, Jeremy, 1994, "The Classics and New Poetry", *The Classical Journal*, 40:77–91.
36 Steiner, George, 1967, *Language and Silence*, London: Faber & Faber, p. 309.
37 For example: Durrell, Lawrence, 1980a, *Collected Poems, 1931–1974*, ed. James A. Brigham. London: Faber & Faber.
38 For example: Durrell, Lawrence, 1952b, *Sappho*, London: Faber & Faber.
39 For example: Durrell, Lawrence, 1974b, *The Best of Antrobus*, London: Faber & Faber.
40 For example: Durrell Lawrence, 1957b, *Bitter Lemons*, London: Faber & Faber.
41 Durrell, Lawrence, 1952a, *A Key to Modern British Poetry*, London: Peter Neville.
42 Begnal, Michael H., 1990, *On Miracle Ground*, London: Associated University Press, pp. 23–56.
43 Durrell, Lawrence, 1987, "Letters to T. S. Eliot", *Twentieth Century Literature*, 33/3:348–358.
44 Sligh, Charles, 1998, "Reading the Divergent Weave: A Note and Some Speculations on Durrell and Cortázar", *Deus Loci*, 6:113–118.
45 Pine, Richard, 2005, *Lawrence Durrell: The Mindscape*, Corfu: Durrell School of Corfu.
46 Clawson, James M., 2016, *Durrell Re-read: Crossing the Liminal in Lawrence Durrell's Major Novels*, Maryland: Fairleigh Dickinson University Press.
47 Eagleton, Terry, 1998, "Supreme Trickster", *The New Statesman*, April 24, pp. 48–49.
48 Green, Peter, 1998, "A Small Blond Firework", *The New Republic*, September 14, pp. 55–60.
49 Durrell, Sappho, 1991, "Journals and Letters", in *The Family: They Fuck You Up*, London: Granta, pp. 55–92.
50 Robson, Barbara, 1991, "The Darker Side of Durrell", *The Sunday Telegraph*, May 26, pp. 23–26.
51 MacNiven, Ian S., 2005, "Lawrence Durrell", in *The Oxford Dictionary of National Biographies*, Oxford: Oxford University Press, pp. 324–330.
52 I participated in the Centenary conference held in London in June 2012.
53 For further details about past and current activities of the Library, refer to the Library's website: www.durrelllibrarycorfu.org, where updated information is provided.
54 A concise summary of the plot is provided in the next chapter, p. 40.

1

PSYCHOANALYSIS, WRITING AND EXILE

In this chapter, I will explore the theoretical assumptions that my study of the *Quartet* is based upon. Naturally, there are many theoretical angles one could adopt when dealing with literature. As I will show later, it is not my intention to make the picture (the *Quartet*) fit the frame (theory) but rather to show how psychoanalytic insights helped me to read and understand the *Quartet*.

The Alexandria Quartet explores the contradictory views that different narrative perspectives offer of the same events, united in the single goal, as expressed by Darley in the opening pages of *Justine*, to turn the key of memory within him through the laborious and treacherous act of writing.[1] The different narrative voices in the four volumes of the *Quartet* form a multi-layered literary landscape, where the identity and significance of the protagonists changes at different key points in the plot.[2]

Durrell's choice of polyphonic narratives is a key element in his seemingly post-romantic outlook on reality. Through his writing, he launches on a journey of finding personal happiness and seeking the meaning of life and love in art. In the introduction to *Balthazar*, the second volume of the *Quartet*, he writes that the main concern of the tetralogy is to conduct an investigation into what he initially describes as *modern love*.[3] As the text unfolds, the theme of love changes in nature and reveals raw sexuality underneath, emerging as a contradiction to what had been told up to that point. The contradiction is not resolved, and the paradoxical and ambivalent experiences are present throughout this work as a statement about modern existence. Each one of the four volumes of the tetralogy offers a different narrative of almost the same chain of events, each one dispelling the veracity of the preceding one.[4] As the *Quartet* progresses, the question *what is truth?* still resonates but seems to become marginal, only to make way for other more pertinent questions: *in what way are these stories told*, and *what are the different meanings they sustain?* These questions addressed in the book focus on the different strategies employed to present the different narratives of the plot, signifying the complex nature of the human mind.

The novel is written in the rich and beautiful language Durrell was known for. In the opening pages of *Justine*, a reference is made to the linguistic splendours found only in the depths of the ocean.[5] The metaphor of the ocean echoes the use Freud made of such a metaphor in his communication with the French writer Romain Rolland (1866–1944). Rolland wrote to Freud a letter regarding the limitless, preverbal experience that describes the relation of the individual to this world. In his 1930 essay, *Civilization and Its Discontents*, Freud refers to the letter exchange where they discussed Freud's views on religion. Freud's view of religion as an infantile wish did not prevent him from recognising the "feeling which he would like to call a sensation of 'eternity,' a feeling as of something limitless, unbounded – as it were, 'oceanic'."[6] The allusion suggested in the word *oceanic*, both in the sense that Freud and Rolland give it and in *Justine*, will emerge in subsequent chapters where I discuss the term *the Heraldic Universe* Durrell coined to describe his relation to the world. The mysterious, enigmatic and *unheimliche* nature of the relation of the individual to the world, as perhaps contained in the single word *oceanic*, is a key element in the *Quartet*. Durrell's personal roots, having been born in India and spent his life searching for a place he could call home, were manifested in his sense of not-being-there which he investigated through his writing. His quest for home can be viewed as the search not necessarily for the lost home but rather, as Harold Bloom suggested, as the quest for the place one already inhabits, which is the hardest quest of them all.[7]

The biographical and fictional elements in literature

The interpretation of literature creates a unique meeting place where the biographical and the fictional elements converge. It is true that sometimes the biographical information about the author, for example, proves more dominant than the fiction he created, while at others, the opposite proves right and the work of fiction can be read with no prior knowledge of its biographical origin. Most interesting interpretations of texts offer some combination of the two, and it is hard to imagine the utter absence of either element from any literary analysis. Any attempt to present biographical details as purely objective data, devoid of fictional manipulation, ignores the fact that language is always a fictional and deliberate, albeit often unconscious, act of creativity.

The Alexandria Quartet was written as a work of fiction, but like any piece of text, it is not detached from the actual experiences of its author. I suggest reading, interpreting and analysing the *Quartet* in a manner that recognises the interconnectivity and inseparability of the two elements, so as to enable an understanding of its deepest layers, offering a view into the author's quest for meaning. As Pursewarden, one of the protagonists in *Balthazar* and often Darley's alter-ego, as I will show in subsequent chapters, suggested, we cannot rely on facts to be solid evidence of anything real or tangible, and yet we must still pursue our quest for the truth and accept that our human imagination feeds of reality and creates it at the very same time.[8]

The Israeli scholar Avi Sagi, in his study of Aharon Appelfeld's (1932–2018) *Poland, A Green Land*, elaborated on the complexity of the relations between the biographical and fictional elements in literature, particularly in literature that explores the existential questions at the foundation of the individual seeking his place in the universe.[9] Sagi pointed to the apparent contradiction of these two concepts. While the biographical tale pertains to the life events of the author, its fictional counterpart refers to the written evidence of his consciousness. But this contradiction flounders when we consider that an autobiographical story is also a fictional story, by the fact that both use language, which in turn represents traces of fickle and fallible human memory. Every choice of incorporating a particular detail into a biographical story entails fictionalisation, with connections forged that may not have been present in reality. Once we recount the past, our consciousness is part and parcel of the narrative and a fictional element is embedded into the story.

The denial of the significance and validity of the biographical elements in literary analysis is represented by philosophers such as the French philosopher Roland Barthes (1915–1980), who announced the death of the author, and exiled the biographical elements to the margins.[10] Such a view, denying the significance of the biographical elements of the author for the interpretation and understanding of his work, presumes that the text may be fully read and understood without any context. Such an unequivocal ruling was, in part, a reaction to the psychoanalytic practice of an excessive engagement with the biography of the author, as well as with facile psychologising analysis of the work and the writer's relation to his characters.

On the other hand, the traditional psychoanalytic position assigned a central role to the biographical elements in understanding the text, and relied on psychological analysis of the character of the author to illuminate the text itself. Trying to trace biographical data in the text implies viewing it as personal testimonies containing hints of past events. One of the proponents of such an approach was Marie Bonaparte (1882–1962), a psychoanalyst and a disciple of Freud.[11] She maintained that literary works should be interpreted by analysing the biography of the author.[12] She based her conviction on the classic psychoanalytic view that saw the psychosexual development of the child as the key to understanding the psyche and behaviour of the adult. To understand the literary work fully, the author's sexual development should be traced and deciphered. She proposed to search the text for vestiges of the repressed, censured and forgotten childhood sexuality, in order to interpret the plot and characters. She claimed that the same defensive mechanisms that were at play in the unconscious could also be found in the text. She cited four such mechanisms: *representation*, *condensation*, *splitting* and *displacement*. Such a view of the text, rummaging for traces of the childhood of the author, attracted fierce criticism of the method as a whole. Nevertheless, it still has its merits when one considers the importance of regarding and appreciating the text in its own specific and very particular cultural and biographical context. Disregarding the context and reading the "pure" text can create tunnel vision and lead to an impoverishment of the text itself. We cannot therefore ignore the various contexts that attend the reality in which the work was written.

Such was the view of one of the earliest hermeneutic philosophers, Friedrich Schleiermacher (1768–1834), who wrote as early as the eighteenth century that: "The Particular can be understood only from the Whole."[13] Individuals can be understood only in their particular historical context. Psychoanalytic analysis of texts offers more than the hermeneutic understanding of the cultural and historical context. Nor does it limit itself to searching for expressions of repressed sexuality in a text. Psychoanalytic interpretation may suggest an unconscious conceptual framework of the text which can be inspiring and suggestive for the reader without reducing the original text to a mere screen that conceals the details of the repressed childhood of the writer. Scrupulous use of psychoanalytic conceptualisations can incorporate the understanding of biographical elements to deepen the understanding of fictional elements of the work and clarify their congruence. To cite the contemporary hermeneutic philosopher thinker Hans-Georg Gadamer (1900–2002), literary analysis deals with the questions found in the actual text so as to dwell on their meaning: "Thus a person who wants to understand must question what lies behind what is said . . . we can understand a text only when we have understood the question to which it is an answer."[14] The text can be understood only once the question it seeks to address is clarified.

Combining the fictional and biographical elements lends weight to the reflective process that the reader is engaged in while reading. In the words of literary critic Norman Holland (born 1927):

> Like every human experience, literature has both something subjective in it and something objective. If we treat "objective" and "subjective" as two neat little boxes and insist on sorting aspects of experience into one or the other, we shall have no way of accounting for literary creation or re-creation, or all the other kinds of total experience that combine the two . . . the problem, then, is not to sort out subjective from objective but to see how the two combine when we have experiences.[15]

Reading the *Quartet* as a work of fiction while being aware of the biographical elements that are intertwined into the narrative is the very process that allows us to follow the existential journey undertaken by Durrell as a writer. *The Alexandria Quartet* can be read independently of the biographical details of the life of Lawrence Durrell and be greatly enjoyed and appreciated for its rich language and original ideas. However, such a reading might be amiss, as it will overlook the cultural context that inspired the work. Lawrence Durrell wrote the *Quartet* during a definite period in history, at a particular point in his life. As Mikhail Bakhtin (1895–1975) wrote:

> The author of the work is only present in the work as a whole, and in none of the moments of this whole individually, least of all in its content as detached

> from this whole. He dwells in that moment that is indiscernible from the whole, where form and content merge inextricably, and it is in the form that he is most palpable to us . . . the real author cannot become a character, as he is the creator of each and every character, of everything that is simile in the work. What is referred to as the "author's character" can only be a character in the work at hand (which is indeed a special kind of character). The painter often paints himself in the picture (at its margin), as well as painting his self-portrait. But we do not see the author per se in the self-portrait (he himself cannot be seen), no more than we can see him in any other work by the author at hand, anyway; more than anywhere else, he is revealed to us in the most exquisite paintings . . . we only see the artist in his work, but never outside thereof.[16]

The Alexandria Quartet calls for a painstaking, careful interpretation of the complex fabric where fictional and biographic elements interweave. As literary critic Shoshana Felman (born 1924) and psychoanalyst Dori Laub wrote in their book *Testimony*:

> Far from simply represented or reflected, biography and history are rewritten, translating one another into text in a way that sees them both rethought. To get to the bottom of the context's effect on the text, we must not only know the context, the empirical association – we must also learn to read it: parallel to the text and as part thereof. We shall therefore seek to show how the perfectly obvious, legitimate, critical call for a contextualization of the text – should itself, at the same time, undergo exposure to a process that is not as familiar (but every bit as essential), which is the textualisation of the context.[17]

The *Quartet* is not an autobiography, but as Durrell made a clear effort to imbue the novel with details one can identify as belonging to his own biography and person, it is wise to consider the term coined by Guillaume Lejeune, *the thing beyond*, as the horizon where the author of the work and the narrator converge. I would argue that as such, this work of fiction is a testimony to Durrell's literary life project.[18] One example for such a convergence is the name of the *Quartet*'s main narrative voice and protagonist, L.G. Darley, which is almost identical to the author's name, L.G. Durrell.[19] Almost too obvious, this phonetic affinity attests to Durrell's ironic designs. On the one hand, it does point to the play between the biographical and fictional elements in the work, but, on the other, creates a certain distance and perhaps alerts readers from falling into the trap of facile psychologising analysis.[20]

Freud discussed the conscious and unconscious aspects of choosing a name for a literary protagonist in reference to the biography of the author in his seminal work on dreams.[21] Freud suggested that the appearance of similarity in names between literary characters and their authors is a symptom of *hysterical identification* and an effort to engage in mental processing of painful emotional experiences, like personal loss. Freud based his observation on *Hamlet* and suggested that the choice of the name of the anguished prince reflected a reconstruction of the psychic pain William Shakespeare (1564–1616) experienced in relation to the deaths of his father and son, Hamnet. Hamnet Shakespeare (1585–1596) died when he was eleven years old just before the estimated time that Shakespeare wrote *Hamlet*. His father, John Shakespeare (c.1531–1601), died at the very same period during which the play was being written. As the play deals with complex father-son-ghost relationships, it is clear how Freud noted the striking similarity between Hamlet and Hamnet and attributed unconscious motives to the choice of the name of protagonist. He claimed that the choice of the name and the plot can be attributed to the effort made by Shakespeare to reinstate his son's memory and deal with the grief over his and his father's deaths.

The quest for reinstating the lost object of a painful emotional experience can be found early in *Justine*, the first volume of the *Quartet*. Darley recounts that he is embarking on the journey of writing in order to come to grips with the burden of the past, with all that he has been through and has driven him to his temporary exile in the Greek island where he had fled. He hopes he can shake free of his existential pain with the help of writing, yet acknowledges that it may not have the desirable healing effect. He nevertheless hopes that words can revive his memories and convey some of his existential experience. Even if he fails to reach the point where pain becomes art, he nevertheless cannot abandon the effort.[22] *The Alexandria Quartet* is the author's attempt at processing a primeval emotional experience by bringing together the fictional and biographical elements. Later, I will describe this experience as *the secret wound*, a term I borrow from the work of the French-Bulgarian psychoanalyst and philosopher Julia Kristeva (born 1941) on exile and strangeness.[23] The present work will focus on a synchronic study of some aspects of the life of Lawrence Durrell and some of his work, in particular *The Alexandria Quartet* and some of his letter correspondence. Durrell, of course, continued to write profusely during the thirty odd years after the *Quartet*'s publication, but the scope of this book does not allow a serious study of his later works.

Before embarking on this journey, and since this book is also written for those who have not yet read the *Quartet*, I will briefly outline the book's main plot points so that uninitiated readers can be given a map to guide them through the forthcoming labyrinthine voyage. A word of caution is in order, though: this plot summary is a virtual sin, as it sucks out much of the life that pulsates through the *Quartet*. There is absolutely no substitute to reading the *Quartet* itself. Nevertheless, here it is.

The plot

Darley is a teacher of British descent who arrives in Alexandria, under the tutelage of a French diplomat, Pombal. He is in a relationship with Melissa, a local cabaret dancer. During his first year in the city, he meets Justine, the Jewish wife of Nessim Hosnani, a well-to-do Coptic businessman, during a local cultural function, where she seduces Darley and takes him as her lover. At the same time, Nessim befriends Darley for motives that have yet to transpire.

David Mountolive arrives in Egypt as British Ambassador. He becomes close to the Coptic Hosnani family (whom he had known during an earlier posting to Egypt at the start of his diplomatic career when he was also the lover of Leila, Nessim's mother) only to discover the secret plot hatched by Nessim and Justine to increase the political standing of the Coptic minority in Egypt. The plot is based upon the strategic idea of smuggling arms to the Jewish underground in early 1940s Palestine, and thereby striking an alliance between the prospective Jewish state and the Coptic minority, in light of the burgeoning Muslim majority in Egypt. When Mountolive learns of the scheme, he feels torn between his loyalty to Leila, Nessim and Justine, on the one hand, and his allegiance to Britain, on the other.

Aware of the suspicions against Nessim, the writer Pursewarden, a renowned British intellectual, who also works for the diplomatic service in town, struggles to believe him at first and even ends up clashing with Maskelyne, head of the British intelligence service. But with Melissa confirming the rumour as true, he decides to take his own life lest he compromise his standing, as well as fearing his incestuous relationship with his blind sister Lisa is revealed as she begins a relationship with Mountolive.

Darley realises that he has been manipulated by Justine in her attempt to find out whether Pursewarden is aware of their plot and plans to sabotage it. When the scheme is exposed by Mountolive, Justine disappears from Alexandria, after the traditional duck shoot at the lake, where Capodistria, a man familiar to Darley from Justine's accounts of him raping her as a child, is apparently accidentally killed. Nessim manages to avoid arrest with bribes that cost him his entire estate.

Darley leaves Alexandria and moves to another part of Egypt to work as a teacher. Later, after his return to Alexandria, Melissa dies, and he leaves the city again to a remote Greek island, taking Melissa's and Nessim's child with him. Two years later, Dr. Balthazar, a physician, who heads a local Kabballah study group, arrives at the island with his notes of Darley's manuscript. Clea, a local Alexandrian painter, writes Darley a letter, telling him her version of the plot.

Darley then returns to Alexandria where he stays until the end of the war. He meets a devastated Justine and Nessim and forms a romantic relationship with Clea, who has lost her hand in a diving accident. He returns to the Greek island, as he finds himself the beneficiary of Pursewarden's fortune and resolves to dedicate his life to writing.

Psychoanalysis and literature

As George Steiner suggested, the study of language is central to both psychoanalysis and literature: "The raw material and instrumentality of Freudian analysis are semantic."[24] The study of language as a means of understanding human consciousness is a pillar of contemporary psychoanalytic theory. Shoshana Felman places the two, literature and psychoanalysis, as sibling disciplines.[25] Psychoanalytic theory is therefore not an exclusive authority in the study of the literary object. Both literature and psychoanalysis observe human consciousness through its reflection in human behaviour and especially language.

One particular field where psychoanalysis and literature share interest is dreams. The interpretation of dreams as textual material that has both manifest and latent layers is an example of the vicissitudes of the common playground of literature and psychoanalysis. In chapter three I will explore dream and dream work further, but it is important at this early stage to note the distinction between the dream itself (the text) and the dream-analysis (textual interpretation). Freud presumed the existence of an unconscious region of the mind, which mainly comprises repressed sexual phantasies. These fantasies seek their way out into the conscious mind and can be detected through the construction of the dream-as-text. Their appearance in the dream is mediated and censured so that their linguistic expressions are governed by a complex system of filters (defences), whereby its meanings are altered, constructed and re-constituted. These defences use strategies such as *displacement, condensation, screen memory, sublimation* and *projection* to distort the original meaning. In the analysis of the dream-as-text, these defences need to be observed and worked over to allow the interpretive process to unfold. An interpretation that relies on such a psychoanalytic method allows a particular reading of the text, echoing the work of the psychoanalyst who listens to the patient's unconscious contents as they appear in the telling of the dream and during the therapeutic hour. At this point, a reminder may be necessary that the analogy between textual interpretation and clinical interpretation can only go so far; by no means can it extend to equating therapy with writing/reading, though both, of course, can have beneficial and enlightening consequences for the individuals involved.

The connection between psychoanalytic theory and the study of literature dates back to the early days of psychoanalytic theory and reflects the cultural background that Freud lived in. His classic education and the influences of German romanticism in his youth meant that literature was a source of inspiration for his ideas, as well as serving him with an arena to examine the validity of his ideas in his quest for a scientific base for his theories.[26] Freud was acquainted, and corresponded, with contemporary writers, like Rainer Maria Rilke (1875–1926), Thomas Mann (1875–1955), Arthur Schnitzler (1862–1931) and Stefen Zweig (1881–1942), and his writing was inspired by writers like Johann Wolfgang von Goethe (1749–1932), Friedrich Schiller (1759–1805) and William Shakespeare. He used his analytic methods to interpret literary works so as to elaborate and demonstrate his ideas. In 1897, Freud performed the first psychoanalytic study of a text by the Swiss poet C. F. Meyer (1825–1898), claiming to have uncovered the poet's repressed memory of a liaison with his sister.[27] Freud was excited about the prospect of wielding psychoanalytic tools to analyse literary characters and pursued it throughout his career.[28] He thought poetry and literature were even better positioned to reveal the innermost truthful nature of human beings than his own psychoanalytic theories, and argued that his earlier studies into hysteria and neurosis could be treated as short stories.[29] He thought that the writer was an individual who had succeeded in transforming and sublimating his unconscious (sexual) phantasies without disturbing his mental balance. The writer creates a fictional world which he sets apart from reality. Writing serves as a mental space that glosses over the imperfections of reality.

Later theorists such as L.C. Knights, for instance, concurred and claimed that certain texts hold the potential for mental change.[30] Poems written by poets such as Emily Dickinson (1830–1886), William Blake (1757–1827) and W.H. Auden (1907–1973) can inspire the readers and affect their psyche, both consciously but also through preverbal processes. Reading such texts can have a therapeutic value by allowing sublimative and transformative action to take place. This *modus operandi* of the text is often unintentional on the part of the writers themselves and operates as an imaginary link between the unconscious of the author and the reader.

The aesthetic experience that takes place as we face a piece of art or read a text that inspires us deeply is a complex process that draws on early childhood experiences. This aesthetic experience comprises two levels: on the first level, the reader succeeds in imagining the phantasy offered by the writer as their [the reader's] own. The second level maintains the illusion that the character portrayed by the text is an actual one. It is the readers' ability to contain this complex experience – which rests on their ability to identify – that generates the aesthetic experience. In his later work, psychoanalyst Thomas Ogden (born 1946) explored the affinity between writers and therapists.[31] Ogden, who integrated Freudian thought into later theoretical developments in psychoanalysis, pointed to the similarities between the attention required from the reader and the attention required from the therapist.[32] A parallel can be drawn between how the therapist listens to the patient's words and how the reader reads the text. The therapist follows the patient's words to derive meaning from them – an outcome of the therapeutic situation, which includes not only the verbal content, but also its sensual impact upon the therapist. Similarly, the readers submit themselves to the text's influence. Ogden suggests that the readers, like the patient, do not have to search the text for any latent or 'real' meaning, but rather to immerse themselves in the actual reading experience. Analysing two of Jorge Luis Borges' (1899–1986) poems, Ogden claims that such an immersion generates an emotional experience in the reader and patient alike, allowing them to process significant and even troubling life events such as grief.[33] Reading at times of emotional pain can be an act of creativity that allows the reader to heal and form within themselves the psychic space required for the integration and absorption of the pain into the fabric of their life.

The act of reading can also have a therapeutic outcome, as it encourages readers to identify and understand the protagonist in the text. Once the reader's attention is drawn to the experience of others and finds points of identification with them, he can integrate these experiences into his own. In his study of Albert Camus' (1913–1960) work, Jose Barchilon claims that the novel can be described as a complex symbolical structure designed to restore and create connections between the reader's conscious and unconscious layers. These connections are not unlike the ones restored and created during therapy between the different parts of the self. In therapy and reading alike, connections between different elements, both conscious and unconscious, of the mind are restored. Furthermore, Barchilon makes quite a dramatic claim that these connections amount to cultural and social awakenings that individual readers undergo, and being as they are agents belonging to wider circles, these awakenings have wide social repercussions that can lead to social change.[34]

Another example of psychoanalytic-informed literary analysis can be found in the work of the psychoanalyst Heinz Kohut (1913–1981). Kohut, the founder of the Self psychology school of psychoanalysis, interpreted Thomas Mann's *Death in Venice*. He claimed that the anguish plaguing Mann while writing the novel, because of the suicide of his second sister and his mother's death, informed his creative process while writing his masterpiece. The very act of writing facilitated the *displacement* of the unbearable emotional pain onto the protagonist of the book and thus helped Mann maintain his own mental balance.[35] One could ask – *was that true? Did Mann really do that?* The answer lies in what literary critic Donald Spence argued – once we integrate psychoanalytic insights into literature, the question should be *whether they hold as a convincing narrative rather than as a historical truth*.[36]

If we accept that *narrative truth* is a more adequate term to address these issues, we can accept an argument as made by Andrew Brink in his study of the influence of the Elizabethan poets on the early phase of Durrell's work. Brink claimed that what mostly motivates an author is the sense of inner loss which he tries to repair through his writing. Writing is then perceived to be a restorative process, dealing with depressed aspects of the self, which, in Durrell's case could explain his later preoccupation with his complex and *unheimliche* sense of belonging as a result of his sense of loss of his connection to his birthplace and primeval homeland, India.[37]

Psychoanalytic interpretation and *The Alexandria Quartet*

The assumption that the unconscious processes of the writer are reflected in the form and content of the work itself through projective and sublimative mechanisms is one of the key elements of psychoanalytic-informed interpretations of literary texts. At the beginning of the *Quartet*, Darley writes that his aim in writing this work was to transform personal pain into art, or, in other, Freudian words, to sublimate his personal experiences.[38] A word of caution is in place here, before applying psychoanalytic insights to the reading of the *Quartet*: the present study is no reduction of Durrell's work to a mere psychological analysis of his life. The purpose of psychoanalytic interpretation as a therapeutic practice lies in the psychoanalyst-patient conversations.[39] The application of psychoanalytic textual interpretation methods to literary works does not necessarily translate the therapeutic model into the literary field. The literary text and its narrator are not a patient whose words are given to interpretation. This study will advance in light of Durrell's own words through the lips of Leila, Nessim's mother, when she warned that words are capable of killing love.[40] George Steiner offered a definition of the interpretive process which perhaps can perform the delicate analysis without causing harm:

> An interpreter is a decipherer and communicator of meanings. He is a translator between languages, between cultures and between performative conventions. He is, in essence, an executant, one who 'acts out' the material before him so as to give it intelligible life.[41]

The *Quartet* is by no means unintelligible and does not need anyone's interpretation to give it life. Nevertheless, I do intend my study to be an encounter between two languages, two cultures: that of the words written by Durrell and those written by a few psychoanalytic thinkers. It is a journey in both the worlds of the *Quartet* and of psychoanalysis, a reading, encountering and ingesting of texts so as to make them into a live presence.

The work of Freud and some of his contemporaries engaged Lawrence Durrell throughout his life, offering him a major source of inspiration, in content and structure alike.[42] Durrell's passion to get to the bottom of the latent and manifest processes that had made him the person he had become, led him in the direction of such theories as found in 1930s Europe and later. Freud's ideas of infantile sexuality as a main motivational element in the development of the individual found a receptive ear in Durrell. He was aware of Freud's studies in sexuality and dreams and was inspired by them, even when omitting to reference them directly, or when trying to deny their influence on him. His library contained several English and French editions of Freud's writings, from which he even took the epigraph for the work as a whole, as will be explored in depth in chapter five.[43]

As early as his first letters to Miller in 1936, three years prior to Freud's death in his London exile, Durrell acknowledged the influence Freud had upon his work: "Freud . . . you've made these statements about my absorption of him, and the influence, several times. True, I have read him well."[44] Freud was not the only psychoanalytic influence on Durrell. He also read Freud's disciples, like Otto Rank and Georg Groddeck, who perhaps influenced him even more, at least consciously. It is no wonder therefore that psychoanalytic insights found their way into the *Quartet* itself, alongside camouflaged and semi-camouflaged biographical references to those thinkers. The concept of *screen memory*,[45] for example, referring to the way significant and troubling early memories are often "hidden" behind trivial but persistent later memories, appears explicitly in *Justine*, as Darley describes events which haunt Justine.[46] Other concepts used by Freud such as *misreading* and *slips of the tongue*, are used by Durrell to describe how truth came to light.[47] As well as being a source of inspiration, psychoanalysis also raised resistance in Durrell. This ambivalence found its way into the text itself. He resented attempts to subject his characters to facile psychologising analysis, as in the example where he refuses to describe Justine as nymphomaniac as it would reduce her into a Freudian idea rather than see her as the whole complex and mythical human being that she was, beyond simplistic pigeon-holing.[48] His ambivalence led him to rely on psychoanalytic-informed insights when constructing the complex plot(s) (see chapters two and three), but also planting warning signs throughout the text to caution against over-reliance on those very same insights. Durrell's attitude to psychoanalytic theory is tantamount to his attitude to his actual or imaginary homeland – he drew nearer and further from it by turns, in reality and writing alike – as part of an effort to define his relation to it, time and again.[49]

As will be discussed in chapter four, Durrell spent a lifetime trying to return and restore a sense of belonging which had been perhaps only whole in his birthplace

India. He never returned to India, and developed a complicated inner state of belonging, a form of an imaginary homeland which can be best found in his writing. The process was inexhaustible and for the most part creative. Its goal was not to actually find a place, as he could perhaps have in Britain, the home of his ancestors. It was the voyage itself that inspires him with the illusive sense of meaning he craved. His quest was towards the place of absence and loss that had become his home. He tried to fill that place with words as well as with the gaps between the words, the silence of the solitary artist. That silence is as meaningful as the words that interrupt it. *Justine* ends with a resounding reflection spoken by Darley as he sits down at his desk to begin the process of writing. He turns to the reader and suggests that the success of what he is about to embark upon, and the real difficulty, is in interpreting the silence he feels is surrounding him.[50]

The interpretation of the silence around man is one of the places psychoanalysis seeks to explore in its quest for unconscious meaning. Within that silence, within the unconscious realm of the individual lies the creative kernel of the writer. Freud, in his 1908 essay entitled *Creative Writers and Day-Dreaming*, explores the origins of the inspiration of writers.[51] He makes a distinction between two types of writers: those who derive inspiration from ancient texts, traditions and popular mythologies, and those who seemingly rely on nothing but their own personal experiences. Durrell explores the question of the origins of creativity throughout the *Quartet*, in his quest to trace the inspirations of the different narrators. By so doing, he consigns himself to the latter category defined by Freud. He implies that inspiration lies in the writer's personal experiences and his effort to come to grips with them. Freud wrote that a writer was a man who succeeded in transforming his unconscious childhood phantasies without endangering his mental well-being, the feared consequence of having his repressed conflicts and wishes exposed. Like a child, the writer creates an imaginary world separated from reality. Writing allows the individual to give creative expression to his deepest strata of being, enabling him to work through his inner conflicts. According to Freud, it is an option that was open to every individual: "Every man is a poet at heart."[52] In the *Quartet*, it is not only that every man is a poet, he is also a reader. The *Quartet* is replete with references to the experiences of reading. In fact, The *Quartet* can be described as a series of different readings of the several texts (sometimes even the same texts), which combine together to form the spine of the plot. For Durrell, the process of writing and reading that lies at the work's core is the very thing that spurs the development of the reflective process, which allows his shaping as an artist, as he speaks through the words of Pursewarden, who suggests that the writer needs to refer the reader to search for the blank pages in the novel, thus encouraging them to find their own creativity within the silence that encompasses them.[53] Literature and psychoanalysis, respectively, can set off a reflective process in the reader/author and the therapist/patient. The blank page cited by Durrell is not necessarily the *blank screen* referred to by Freud in his recommendations to the psychoanalyst, but a parallel can indeed be drawn between the two concepts.[54] The reflective process calls on the author/reader and therapist/patient to venture deep inside their consciousness, silences and memories, and with the help of language – written, read or spoken – to set out on a quest for meaning in life.

Trying to understand a literary character, whether it is the narrator, protagonist or any other figure in the book, is unlike trying to understand real flesh and blood individuals.[55] The literary character created in the writing process is a reflective expression and a product of the imagination of the author, allowing us to interpret it without stepping into psychologising. What we are interpreting in fact is the reflective process of the author. The interpretation offered to the *Quartet*'s characters, therefore, has Lawrence Durrell's reflective process in mind. The characters he created can be seen, as Darley himself says in relation to Justine, not as real people but more as literary references, notes made upon reading a poem. Darley even suggests that perhaps all human contacts are merely reflections of our attempts to construct them through words, rather than actual, tangible exchanges. We see what we want to see in the people that surround us. They are as real, or imaginary, as figures in a novel.[56]

One of the important psychoanalytic developments that followed and deepened the work of Freud was the Austrian psychoanalyst Melanie Klein (1882–1960).[57] In her theory, which was based upon clinical experiences with children, she developed the notion that we deal with the real world only through our internalised vision of it. This internal vision, *object relations*, is a dynamic system which is nourished by and informs our perceptual presence in the world. So when Darley wonders whether his relation to Justine is a real one or one which he has constructed based upon her internalised image in his mind, he is touching upon a central issue in psychoanalytic theory.

Another key concept that can be read in the *Quartet* through psychoanalytic glasses is sexuality as a driving force of personal and interpersonal development. The inspiration Durrell drew from Freudian theory regarding the centrality of sexuality and the damage wreaked when it is suppressed is poignantly evident throughout the work. Pursewarden, again in the role of Darley's superego, writes in his suicide letter that sex equals culture. The truth about human motives is to be found through the investigation of the way through which their sexuality appears and drives their actions at different points in time.[58] Pursewarden's words could not better express the central place that sexual development and sexuality hold in Freudian theory. Sexuality, and its sublimated expression in (romantic) love, is considered a motivational drive throughout life.[59] The original Freudian theories have been developed and modified extensively since 1905, not least because of Feminist and Post-Structuralist criticism, as well as new insights gained by modern development in the clinical application of the theories. It is not within the scope of this work to explore these developments in detail; suffice to say that their main premise, at the time when Durrell most likely read them, was that every individual goes through a developmental course where he experienced and processed his relations with others, from birth onwards, through sensual experience that is continually converted into mental structures. Not all of those experiences are remembered or acknowledged. Most are forgotten, repressed, projected and even disavowed as part of the normative process of socialisation. Those experiences sink into our unconscious, where they continue to seek expression. Rather than disappearing, they create mental structures that drive the individual's behaviour to achieve primal satisfaction and its sublimated derivatives, like politics and art. In chapter four, I will expand upon the way Durrell explored sexuality in the *Quartet*, either as a stage where the protagonists pursue their search for happiness and love, or as the hidden and repressed labyrinthine workings of their tormented souls.

Belonging and exile – was Durrell an exile?

Durrell had his first taste of exile at eleven, when he was sent away from his native India to England for his education. For the rest of his life Durrell would go back to this time, citing it as a key to his existential experience of being away from his home – which left a mark of sadness and loneliness but also played a role in his formation as a writer. One could speculate that the link between exile and writing was first established in Durrell's mind when his father asked him what he wanted to become, and answered that he wanted to be a writer. His reply resulted in him being sent to England, under the pretext of providing him with the intellectual and cultural setting to realise his wish. This link between exile and writing, wrapped up in the father's part-wish part-command, would become a haunting presence in Durrell's life.

Durrell's definition as an exiled author stretches the limits of this term beyond its immediate concrete meaning. Unlike authors like Vladimir Nabokov, Samuel Beckett (1906–1989), Joseph Conrad (1857–1924) and others, who had physically left their countries *and* mother tongue to write in a foreign language, Durrell wrote almost entirely in his native English and never even tried to return to India, his birthplace. For Durrell, the issue of the relation to a home is seized with complexities. I have suggested earlier that the Freudian term *unheimliche* is perhaps the most appropriate to describe that relation.

Durrell indeed moved between quite a staggering number of places in his lifetime – India, England, Corfu, mainland Greece, Rhodes, Cyprus, Egypt, Argentina, Yugoslavia and France – quite a whirlwind that could unsettle anyone's relation to his home even with a more secure base. Even a cursory glance at Durrell's biography would reveal that he was not actually exiled from any of those countries, with the exception of his departure from India as a child and, later, when forced to leave Greece during the Second World War. To earn the title *exiled writer*, one needs to feel in relation to one specific country that can be called home. Did Durrell have a home in that sense? Designating one of these places as Durrell's homeland proves an impossible undertaking. Is it not more accurate to say that the frequent moves he made since the age of eleven made him a man in whose world the homeland functioned not as an actual place to return to but rather a place to seek? Durrell was content to inhabit whichever place would afford him a setting convenient enough for writing. In this sense, writing was his motherland, while he himself embodies Jacques Derrida's (1930–2004) statement that "language is the homeland."[60] In chapter five, I will argue that in Greece, young Durrell found a location nearest to a place he could call home where he established his authentic voice as a writer. He found the geographic climate agreeable, while the cheap livelihood and social surroundings provided the setting he required to write. The advent of the Second World War forced him into a series of transitions to places he experienced as foreign. Was it thus that he had earned his status as an exile writer? Only during the late 1950s did he eventually come again upon his sought-after conditions in the south of France, which he was no longer willing to leave, even when he had the wherewithal to live wherever he chose. For Durrell, home was where he was able to immerse himself in the business of writing.

I suggest that *The Alexandria Quartet* can be read as an exploration of the relation between the individual, the place he inhabits and the place he has lost. It is in this context that the laden, complex concepts of *belonging* and *exile* should be examined. One's homeland can therefore be thought of as *The Other* and seen in the light of the words of Pursewarden, who claimed that the real Other was the one found within one's self.[61] The search for one's homeland is the search for one's self, and as such can be described only as an ongoing process, which can end only in death.

Everybody has a significant relation with the place they inhabit at a given moment. Generally speaking, this relation is taken for granted by most people most of the time. Most people feel secure enough where they are to not make an issue of it. It is only at certain times in one's life, through personal change or crises or through social upheavals, that the relation between the individual and his home comes to the front of his awareness. It is at those moments that attention needs to be given to maintain and even repair that relation. It is at those moments that the individual realises that what he thought of as natural and trivial is in fact far from it. These moments of change are also moments of loss. As Roland Barthes wrote in his seminal work *Mythologies* (1972): "I had time to experience both a sense of familiarity and one of alienation, measuring stability against change, past against present tense."[62] The experience of loss is dealt with differently by different people, depending on many variants such as their cultural background, financial and familial stability and many more. The writer can deal with such moments through writing and thus give room for the process of adjustment and even grief to take place.

The moment when the homely, *Heimlich*, becomes unsafe and strange, *unheimliche*, is seminal to modern culture. As the Indian writer Homi Bhabha (born 1949) wrote, that which is lost, that which was familiar, makes way for the new, which is in fact a hybrid of old and new.[63] Such a change not only needs to occur as a result of a personal or social calamity. Our view of what is familiar can change through reflection and insights. Thus, our recollection of a childhood memory can change and have different meanings attributed to it, either as a result of new insight or through new information. That process was called by Freud *nachträglich*, a change in our recollection of the past which now seems as true as the previous one did earlier, prior to the change. This is quite common in therapy. And this is what can happen when we use writing, as Durrell did, in order to restore our sense of self, to deal with an experience of loss, as he did in his relation to his home. The Israeli photographer and philosopher Ariella Azoulay (born 1962) described in her analysis of Walter Benjamin's (1892–1940) essay, *The Work of Art in the Age of Mechanical Reproduction* (1936), such a moment whereby the original place changes its value due to our reflective process. She describes the loss of the place as "a transition from a unique place, which has to be attended if it is to be experienced, to a place that, thanks to the different reproduction technologies, can be experienced without our presence therein."[64] The *reproduction technology* in this case is the process of writing through, which Durrell tried to return to. That unique place in the present case is Durrell's homeland. What is that homeland in this case? Is it his birthplace in India? As I have written, Durrell kept a longing attitude towards that place, describing it as the lost Eden, to which it is no longer possible to return. Is it London, where he spent his formative years but hated every minute of it?

In *Mountolive*, Durrell speaks through the lips of the diplomat Mountolive, who describes his periodical return to London as a return to a beloved person as he was returning to a place of interrogation. He returns to the sense of melancholy which he loves and hates at the same time. London feels like a tomb, a tomb he belongs to, a tomb where sexuality and eccentricity flourish. It is a home he does not want to be a part of.[65] Durrell could not return physically to a place where he could feel at home since that inner space was too hurt to accommodate such a return. It was only through writing that he could try to return and restore himself. As I will suggest in chapter four, it was in Alexandria, the city of memory, that Durrell set the scene for this attempt to recapture his lost sense of belonging. The city of Alexandria offered Durrell a poetic breadth and platform for his inner mental processes, described in his letters from his time there. In the *Quartet* itself, exile is described as a state that even the local people of Alexandria cannot escape, given the many historic upheavals that have befallen the city and made it unrecognisable even to them. The state of exile is no mere outcome of one historical crisis or another. Nor is it a reflection of some cultural transformation, but rather the fundamental state of the city, which casts its shadow on all its inhabitants. Being in Alexandria is being in exile.[66]

Alexandria as portrayed in *The Alexandria Quartet* was Durrell's *liminal space*, where he tried to perform the impossible feat of return.[67] This notion of a territory of belonging, that is not necessarily geographic, is consistent with an ambivalent and ambiguous view of one's belonging to one's homeland. It is a view that does not allow for a coherent, essentialist statement on the individual-homeland relation, but rather reveals a coil of complex relations.

The exiled writer

The exiled writer is a specimen of modern Western culture. He carries his inner foreignness in the form of language itself. Andrew Gurr, in his study of exile as it appears in the works of Katherine Mansfield (1888–1923), James Joyce and W.S. Naipaul (born 1932), wrote that "Exile creates the kind of isolation . . . the normal role of the modern writer is to be an exile."[68] For most exiles, the experience is fraught with actual physical misery and hardship. The exile of an African fugitive who flees a hostile regime in search of political asylum in a foreign country is in a different category from the exile of a writer who leaves his home as part of his inner voyage. It is the experience of the individual in the second category that is the subject of this study.

The exile experience as an existential state can be attributed to an individual, a group of people or even to different parts of the same individual. Exile can be studied in social, cultural, psychological and religious contexts.[69] Ella Belfer, for example, describes the collective identity of the Jewish people as essentially based upon the exile experience.[70] Exile itself is not a transitional state of the Jewish people, but rather a profound manifestation of their essence, or in Haviva Pedaya's words: "Being scattered is the primal Jewish myth of existence."[71]

Tracing the development of the category of exile as it appears in literature is a voyage through Western culture.[72] Exile can never be a beneficial experience. It is a calamitous experience leaving in its wake traumatic symptoms that can then be traced through the testimonies of those who survived it.[73] Though not the sole preserve of writers, it is they who mostly leave behind a written testimony of the exile. Michael Seidel introduced the term *exilic imagination* to show that separation from a homeland was tantamount to separation from what the writer's mind was full of.[74] The writer's attempt to return to his home is performed through the act of writing, an effort that by its very nature cannot amount to an actual return, but rather to a linguistic realisation. The homeland experience is perceived as oppressive, hindering total engagement with the creative work, while life in exile can produce better creative conditions. On the other hand, exile separates the writer from his primeval existential conditions, the actual fountain of his work.

Gareth Griffiths studied English-writing by African and Caribbean writers and described a state of *a double exile*, of writers who are away from their native home and culture and write in a language other than their mother tongue.[75] Griffiths showed how this situation can be a catalyst rather than inhibitor for the creative process. He maintained that the work of exiled writers possessed an added value due to the uniqueness of their position of having to translate themselves in order to write. Jacques Derrida described the writer's distance from his culture as a liberating element. Being a foreigner in his own homeland, the individual can pose questions that defy traditional perceptions.[76] Derrida ties these questions to the exclusion of whatever is perceived as an exception and as foreign by society. He draws a direct link between the fact of foreignness, exile and displacement and the use of one's mother tongue:

> What in fact does language name, the so-called mother tongue, the language you carry with you, the one that also carries us from birth to death? Doesn't it figure the home that never leaves us? The proper or property, at least the *fantasy* of property that, as close as could be to our bodies, and we always come back there, would give place to the most inalienable place, to a sort of mobile habitat, a garment or a tent? Wouldn't this mother tongue be a sort

> of second skin you wear on yourself, a mobile home? But also an immobile home since it moves around with us?[77]

Kim Parker, when studying the work of the Croatian writer Dubravka Ugrešić (born 1949), described the state of exile as enriching, as it provided writers with a perspective on their natural cultural habitat, assuming the writer has such a natural habitat in the first place.

As a part in the Anglo-Indian community since the nineteenth century, Durrell's habitat was fragmented to begin with. His sense of belonging was affected by his own distance from that habitat, sending him on a lifetime quest for a new – or re-found – sense of belonging. The exile experience became his *unheimliche* sense of belonging. Having returned to Alexandria and meeting broken Nessim, Darley describes his sense of belonging like a castaway on a familiar coast. Being home feels like a castaway in a place which was meant to embrace him.[78]

Despite the mounting argument that exiled authors reach deep into the creative well, and while their testimonies can be the basis of literary masterpieces, it is also true to say that no geographical exile is required to unleash the powers of imagination. Many other magnificent literary masterpieces that explore deep experiences of estrangement have been written by writers like Marcel Proust or Fernando Pessoa (1888–1935), who never left their homeland, or wandered too far away from it. The sense of estrangement that is perhaps a prerequisite for the inner voyage that writers undertake can, and often does, occur within one's homeland.

Finally, as Zygmunt Bauman (1925–2017) stated, *exile* in contemporary culture is a metaphor for the voyage and encounter with all that is unfamiliar, with the new and the different, within and without.[79] Exile holds the prospect of change and self-discovery. The exiled writer is a person who creates a new cultural experience in exile, in what amounts to creating an imaginary homeland that maintains affinity both with the original culture and host culture. In the *Quartet* itself, exile is described as a state that even the local people of Alexandria cannot escape, given the many historic upheavals that have befallen the city and made it unrecognisable even to them. The state of exile is no mere outcome of one historical crisis or another. Nor is it a reflection of some cultural transformation, but rather the fundamental state of the city, which casts its shadow on all its inhabitants.[80] Exile is both a question mark posed concerning one's sense of belonging and an existential solution to the lost individual. This binary sense is at the very core of the *Quartet*.

The fragmented nature of the exiled writer

The Black Book (1938), Durrell's first book to receive critical acclaim, is the story of a writer who is away from his homeland and culture.[81] It recounts debasing experiences that plunge the protagonist into existential despair, reflected, among other things, in his negative outlook on the culture from which he has fled. The novel is Durrell's early treatment of his testimony on the exile experience. This testimony portrays the subject as a downcast individual. Exile is no cathartic or insight-evoking experience. As George Orwell, Durrell's contemporary (and incidentally, another writer born in India), wrote, exile is a morally demeaning experience and cannot yield fine literature.[82] In his essay on Durrell's close friend, Henry Miller, Orwell found exile detrimental to writers more than to any other artist. Placing language above all as the ultimate expression of all human experience, Orwell thought that the writer's language suffered a mortal blow in exile, as the writer was detached from all those fountains of inspiration and nourishment at his disposal back in the homeland. This mortal blow to the writer's identity while in exile is clearly reflected in how Durrell built the different voices of the narrators in *The Alexandria Quartet*. As discussed in the next chapter, the narrator of the work is not a single voice but rather a fragmented figure, or figures, composed of multiple identities.

The idea of the self as a fragmented entity can be found later, in the work of Julia Kristeva, who maintained that the individual's sense of identity is no solid, uniform verifiable entity, but rather an identity established through the subject's different linguistic, social and psychoanalytical readings. For Kristeva, the discussion about the identity of the subject entails a discussion about language:

> We are no doubt permanent subjects of a language that holds us in its power. But we are subjects in process, ceaselessly losing our identity, destabilized by fluctuations in our relations to the other, to whom we nevertheless remain bound by a kind of homeostasis.[83]

Durrell constructed the voices of the narrator as a figure of destabilised identity made up of multiple selves, with varying ways of constituting himself in different contexts. He thereby positioned him as a postmodern character, plagued with existential questions defining his identity and giving rise to his work. Durrell's narrator is an associative continuum in progress. As the text unfolds, the narrator's identity is equivocal at times, leaving the reader with a sense that he is the narrator of the text he is reading. The narrator is whoever the reader wants him to be.

Finally, the exiled writer who has been able to maintain a sense of his primary affinity to his imaginary or actual homeland does not cease to relate to it, but only realises the prospect of return in his writing and life. The memory of the homeland becomes the return itself, paradoxically allowing the exiled writer to establish a renewed, authentic affinity with his lost homeland. Writing can generate an alternative homeland experience, but it cannot substitute for the actual return. One such example is the work of the Palestinian poet Mahmoud Darwish (1941–2008), most of which was written while he was away from homeland, with exile, longing and return as its central themes. His work is all the more interesting in this context, because even when he was afforded the option of "returning," Darwish took his time accepting it, as the homeland he had been pining for no longer existed. In this sense, the writer's exile is perpetual, the very thing that allows him to write. Return would quell the motivation to write and pose the opposite pole of total dedication to creativity – for which the artist may forego his worldly connections.

Durrell never returned to his geographic homeland of India, but nor did he try to stay in England, which could be thought of as his ancestral and cultural homeland. He spent his life wayfaring from one country to another, only to finally settle down in France, where he completed *The Alexandria Quartet* in 1959, and where died thirty odd years later. He refused British citizenship and was eventually naturalised in France, though this did not put to rest the issues he associated with his sense of belonging. Durrell's sense of belonging was constituted through his writing. *The Alexandria Quartet* was in fact his homecoming, his attempt to search his consciousness for his ties with the place where his subjective identity had been forged. Durrell's return to his homeland played out when he wrote down his experience of belonging to the lost and imaginary homeland.

Notes

1 Durrell, Lawrence, 1957a, *Justine*, London: Faber & Faber, p. 25.
2 The terms "narrator," "author" and "writer" are employed differently throughout the book. To prevent any confusion between the three, let me clarify that "narrator" here denotes any one of the protagonists who recount the tale in the first person voice. "Author" denotes Lawrence Durrell as the author of *The Alexandria Quartet*, with its multiple narrative voices, who himself is present in the work as the overall "owner" of the work. "Writer" denotes the actual Lawrence Durrell, who wrote this work and was, among other things, a native of India who died in France, having been married to four women. The complex relations between these three concepts are explored throughout the book itself.
3 Durrell, Lawrence, 1958a, *Balthazar*, London: Faber & Faber, p. 9.
4 The exception is *Mountolive*, which starts farther back in time than the other three volumes.
5 Durrell, Lawrence, 1957a, *Justine*, London: Faber & Faber, p. 26.
6 Freud, S., 1930, "Civilization and Its Discontents", in J. Strachey, ed., *The Standard Edition of the Complete Psychological Works of Sigmund Freud*, trans. J. Strachey, Vol. XXI, London: Hogarth Press, p. 64.
7 Bloom, Harold, 1997, *The Anxiety of Influence*, New York and Oxford: Oxford University Press.
8 Durrell, Lawrence, 1958a, *Balthazar*, London: Faber & Faber, p. 116. Was Pursewarden a superego, an alter-ego or a double (*Doppelgänger*)? The three terms denote different but related concepts. As the scope of this study is not enough to explore all the subtleties of these terms, I would say that the superego denotes the Freudian notion of a critical internalised psychic agency. The alter-ego and the double refer to a part of the personality which serves as a second, observing version of the self. Freud did refer to the double in his work on *das unheimliche* (*The Uncanny*) as a primal part of the self.
9 Sagi, Avi, 2009, *The Human Voyage to Meaning: A Philosophical-Hermeneutic Study of Literature Works (Hebrew)*, Ramat-Gan: Bar-Ilan University Press, p. 152.
10 Barthes, Roland, 1977, "Death of the Author", in *Image, Music, Text*, trans. Heath Stephen, London: Fontana Press.
11 It was Bonaparte, remote relative of Napoleon Bonaparte, who secured the escape of Freud and most of his family from Nazi occupied Vienna in 1937. She helped Freud to arrive in London and later was instrumental in saving many of his manuscripts and letters. For further details, read: Bertin, Celia, 1983, *Marie Bonaparte: A Life*, London: Quartet Books.
12 Bonaparte, Marie, "The Murders in Rue Morgue", *The Psychoanalytic Quarterly*, 4:259–293.

13 Schleiermacher, Friedrich, 1977, *Two Academy Addresses of 1829: On the Concept of Hermeneutics, Hermeneutics: The Handwritten Manuscripts*, ed., Kimmerle Heinz and trans. Duke James and Forstman Jack, Missoula: Scholar Press, p. 210.
14 Gadamer, Hans Georg, 2004, *Truth and Method*, 2nd Edition, New York: Continuum Press, p. 363.
15 Holland, Norman, H., 1973, *Poems in Person*, New York: W.W. Norton & Company Inc., p. 2.
16 Bakhtin, Michail, 1986, "From Notes Made in 1970–1971", in *Speech Genres & Other Late Essays*, trans. V. Mcgee, Texas: University of Texas Press, p. 195.
17 Felman, Shoshana and Laub Dori, 1992, *Testimony: Crises of Witnessing in Literature, Psychoanalysis and History*, London & New York: Routledge, p. 14.
18 Lejeune, Philippe, 1989, *On Autobiography*, ed., Paul John Eakin and trans. Katherine Leary, Minneapolis: University of Minnesota Press, p. 154.
19 Throughout the novel, Darley's first name is not mentioned but his initials are: L.G. Durrell first names are of course Lawrence George. The fact that Durrell stopped short of using his own full name but only hinted to the initials is another proof of his playfulness in writing
20 Durrell plants several other clues throughout the work that show the affinity he shares with Darley. One example is the citing of protagonist Darley's Irish origins – Durrell's mother too was, according to him, Irish by descent.
21 Freud, S., 1900, *The Interpretation of Dreams: The Standard Edition of the Complete Psychological Works of Sigmund Freud*, ed. J. Strachey and trans. J. Strachey, Vols. IV & V, London: Hogarth Press.
22 Durrell, Lawrence, 1957a, *Justine*, London: Faber & Faber, p. 17.
23 Kristeva, Julia, 1991, *Strangers to Ourselves*, trans. L. S. Roudiez, New York: Columbia University Press.
24 Steiner George, 1978, "A Remark on Language and Psychoanalysis", in *On Difficulty and other Essays*, Oxford: Oxford University Press, p. 48.
25 Felman, Shoshana, 1977, *Literature and Psychoanalysis*, Baltimore and London: The John Hopkins University Press, pp. 12–43; Felman, Shoshana, 2003, *Writing and Madness*, Palo Alto: Stanford University Press, pp. 21–86.
26 Berman, Emanuel, 1993, "Introduction", in Emanuel Berman, ed., *Essential Papers on Literature and Psychoanalysis*, New York and London: New York University Press, pp. 1–15.
27 Gay, Peter, 1990, *Reading Freud*, New Haven: Yale University Press, p. 3.
28 Nägele, Rainer, 1978, *Reading After Freud*, New York: Columbia University Press.
29 Freud, Sigmund and Breuer Joseph, 1893–1895, "Studies on Hysteria", in J. Strachey, ed., *The Standard Edition of the Complete Psychological Works of Sigmund Freud*, trans. J. Strachey, Vol. II, London: Hogarth Press.
30 Knights, L. C., 1980, "Poetry and Things Hard for Thought", *International Review of Psychoanalysis*, 7:125–135.
31 This study culminated in his collaboration in 2013 with his son, the literary critic Benjamin, H. Ogden, in their joint publication, "The Analyst's Ear and the Critic's Ear." Ogden himself published several acclaimed literary works of fiction, *The Parts Left Out* (2014) and *The Hands of Gravity and Chance* (2016), thus crossing the bridge between the two disciplines himself.
32 Ogden, Thomas, 1997, "Some Thoughts on the Use of Language in Psychoanalysis", *Psychoanalytic Dialogues*, 7:1–21.
33 Ogden, Thomas, 2000, "Borges and the Art of Mourning", *Psychoanalytic Dialogues*, 10:65–88.
34 Barchilon, Jose, 1971, "A Study of Camus' Mythpoeic Tale *the Fall* with Some Comments About the Origin of Esthetic Feelings", *Journal of American Psychoanalysis Association*, 19:193–240.
35 Kohut, Heinz, 1957, "*Death in Venice* by Thomas Mann: A Story About the Disintegration of Artistic Sublimation", *Psychoanalysis Quarterly*, 26:206–228.
36 Spence, Donald, 2003, "Listening for Rhetorical Truth", *Psychoanalytical Quarterly*, 83:875–903.

37 Brink, Andrew, 1977, *Loss and Symbolic Repair: A Psychological Study of Some English Poets*, Ontario: The Cromlech Press, pp. 101–142.
38 Durrell, Lawrence, 1957a, *Justine*, London: Faber & Faber, p. 17.
39 There is at least one study that describes a therapeutic use of the insights gained from the *Quartet*. It employs the different narratives of the work as part of a training program for family therapy. For further reading Kaufman, Barbara, 1995, "Training Tales in Family Therapy: Exploring the *Alexandria Quartet*", *Journal of Family and Marital Therapy*, 21:67–81.
40 Durrell, Lawrence, 1958b, *Mountolive*, London: Faber & Faber, p. 48.
41 Steiner, George, 1989, *Real Presences*, London: Faber & Faber, p. 7.
42 Fraser, G. S., 1968, *Lawrence Durrell*, London: Faber & Faber.
43 Durrell had in his library Freud's "The Origins of Psychoanalysis," from which he took the epigraph for *Justine*. The book has many notes made by Durrell in its margins. He also had in his library Freud's 1912a essay, "The Handling of Dream-Interpretation in Psycho-Analysis," and refers to it in his letters to Henry Miller.
44 MacNiven, Ian S., ed. 1988, *The Durrell-Miller Letters, 1935–1980*, London: Faber & Faber, p. 229.
45 Freud, Sigmund, 1899, "Screen Memories", in J. Strachey, ed., *The Standard Edition of the Complete Psychological Works of Sigmund Freud*, trans. J. Strachey, Vol. III, London: Hogarth Press, pp. 299–322.
46 Durrell, Lawrence, 1957a, *Justine*, London: Faber & Faber, p. 81.
47 Freud, Sigmund, 1901, *The Psychopathology of Everyday Live, in the Standard Edition of the Complete Psychological Works of Sigmund Freud*, ed. J. Strachey and trans. J. Strachey, Vol. VI, London: Hogarth Press.
48 Durrell, Lawrence, 1957a, *Justine*, London: Faber & Faber, p. 77.
49 I use the term in the sense given to it by the British-Indian writer, Salman Ahmed Rushdie (born 1941) to denote a home which is not necessarily one's place of birth or a concrete place. Rushdie, Salman, 1991, *Imaginary Homelands: Essays and Criticism 1981–1991*, London: Penguin Books.
50 Durrell, Lawrence, 1957a, *Justine*, London: Faber & Faber, p. 245.
51 Freud, Sigmund, 1908, "Creative Writers and Day-Dreaming", in J. Strachey, ed., *The Standard Edition of the Complete Psychological Works of Sigmund Freud*, trans. J. Strachey, Vol. IX, London: Hogarth Press, pp. 141–154.
52 Ibid., p. 143.
53 Durrell, Lawrence, 1958a, *Balthazar*, London: Faber & Faber, p. 143.
54 In his 1912 essay "Recommendations to Physicians Practising Psycho-Analysis," Freud suggests that when listening to the patient, the therapist should try to listen with evenly suspended attention and empty himself as much as possible of irrelevant thoughts. That concept has been greatly developed in later years and is the current basis for the most important aspect of the therapeutic relationship, i.e. the transference-countertransference paradigm. For further reading: Sandler, Joseph, Dare Christopher and Hope Alex, 1992, *The Patient and the Analyst*, London: Karnac Books.
55 As a clinical social worker practicing psychoanalytic psychotherapy, as well as being a writer, I have been dealing with the tension between clinical and fictional writing throughout my professional life. In a 2016 essay in Hebrew, I have suggested that when a clinician wishes to write upon his professional practice, he should uphold above all the confidence given to him by the patient and never, under any circumstances, divulge any details of the therapy process, even if they are well disguised, as is the common practice. I suggested that the clinician wishing to write can do so by constructing therapeutic tales which are based upon his own subjective experience without referring, implicitly or explicitly, to any patient. Alfandary, Rony, 2016, "To Write or Not to Write: Is That the Question?" *A Therapeutic Tale, Maárg*, 7:1–18.
56 Durrell, Lawrence, 1960, *Clea*, London: Faber & Faber, p. 41.
57 For a thorough survey of the school of Object Relations that Klein is a part of, read Greenberg's and Mitchell's *Object Relations in Psychoanalytic Theory*.

58 Durrell, Lawrence, 1960, *Clea*, London: Faber & Faber, p. 141.
59 Freud, Sigmund, 1905, "Three Essays on Sexuality", in J. Strachey, ed., *The Standard Edition of the Complete Psychological Works of Sigmund Freud*, trans. J. Strachey, Vol. VII, London: Hogarth Press, pp. 125–244.
60 Derrida, Jacques, 2000, *On Hospitality*, trans. Bowlby Rachel, Stanford: Stanford University Press, p. 108.
61 Durrell, Lawrence, 1960, *Clea*, London: Faber & Faber, pp. 98–99.
62 Barthes, Roland, 1972, *Mythologies*, trans. Lavers Annette, New York: The Noonday Press, p. 103.
63 Bhabha, Homi, 1992, "The World and the Home", *Social Text*, 31/32:141–152.
64 Azoulay, Ariella, 2007, *Once Upon a Time: Photography Following Walter Benjamin (Hebrew)*, Ramat-Gan: Bar-Ilan University Press, pp. 56–57.
65 Durrell, Lawrence, 1958b, *Mountolive*, London: Faber & Faber, p. 85.
66 Ibid., p. 147.
67 Turner, Victor, 1969, *The Ritual Process*, New Brunswick and London: Aldine transaction.
68 Gurr, Andrew, 1981, *Writers in Exile: The Identity of Home in Modern Literature*, Sussex, NJ: The Harvester Press and Humanities Press, p. 137.
69 Simpson, John, ed. 1995, *The Oxford Book of Exile*, Oxford and New York: Oxford University Press.
70 Belfer, Ella, 2004, *A Split Identity: The Conflict between the Sacred and the Secular in the Jewish World (Hebrew)*, Ramat-Gan: Bar-Ilan University Press.
71 Pedaya, Haviva, 2011, *Walking Through Trauma: Rituals of Movement in Jewish Myth, Mysticism, and History (Hebrew)*, Tel Aviv: Resling Publishing Ltd., p. 14.
72 Thompson, Edward, 1989, "The Writer in Exile, the Good Years", *Slavic and East European Journal*, 33/4:124–156.
73 Pedaya, Haviva, 2011, *Walking Through Trauma: Rituals of Movement in Jewish Myth, Mysticism, and History (Hebrew)*, Tel Aviv: Resling Publishing Ltd., p. 20.
74 Seidel, Michael, 1986, *Exile and the Narrative Imagination*, New Haven and London: Yale University Press.
75 Griffiths, Gareth, 1978, *A Double Exile*, London: A. Marion Boyar Book, pp. 9–56.
76 Derrida, Jacques, 2000, *On Hospitality*, trans. Rachel Bowlby. Stanford: Stanford University Press.
77 Ibid., pp. 108–109.
78 Durrell, Lawrence, 1960, *Clea*, London: Faber & Faber, p. 31.
79 Bauman, Zygmunt, "Modernity and Ambivalence", in Mike Featherstone, ed., *Global Culture: Nationalism, Globalization and Modernity*, London: Sage, 1990.
80 Durrell, Lawrence, 1958b, *Mountolive*, London: Faber & Faber, p. 147.
81 Durrell, Lawrence, 1938 (1977), *The Black Book*, London: Faber & Faber. The book was first published in 1938 by Obelisk Press in Paris as Faber & Faber refused to publish it in its unexpurgated version. It was then published by Faber & Faber in 1960 in the US. Faber & Faber then published it in Great Britain in 1973. The edition that I have used was published in 1977. I will discuss the book in the final chapter.
82 Orwell, George, 1957, *Inside the Whale*, London: Penguin Books, pp. 9–51.
83 Kristeva, Julia, 1987, *In the Beginning Was Love: Psychoanalysis and Faith*, trans. Arthur Goldhammer, New York: Columbia University Press, p. 40.

2

WHOSE VOICE IS IT ANYWAY? NARRATIVES AND STRUCTURE

The question of the narrative labyrinth created by Durrell, as he attempted a work of multiple meanings that could not be reduced into a simple narrative, is central to the interpretation of the *Quartet*. Durrell created this labyrinth so as to illustrate a certain view of modern life. As Clea says to Darley when she tries to console him through his difficulty in understanding the actions of Justine, no philosophical or psychological theory can contain the full complexity of human experience. We are who we are. The existential questions that we face, the complexities of our relationships and entanglements of our minds – we have to resign ourselves to their enormity and wonder without necessarily making any sense of it.[1]

Most scholars agree that it was the *Quartet*'s complex structure, with its several perspectives and focus on the reflective processes of the different characters, rather than the sexual relationships of the protagonists, that earned it attention and prestige upon its publication. Studies of the structure of *The Alexandria Quartet* have described it as a triptych[2] or palimpsest,[3] and mainly study its labyrinthine nature, the concept of truth and the relation between the dimensions of time and space.[4] Durrell himself stated in 1970 in relation to *Tunc* and *Nunquam* that his characters are simple and one-dimensional, which he then plays with, casting different lights upon them, creating the appearance of depth.[5] Durrell does not suggest an absence of any organising structure for his work. This is not a stream-of-consciousness work, despite its seemingly associative, idiosyncratic continuum. The tetralogy is structured in a manner that attempts to create a literary work that rests on phenomenological approximation to the experience itself. The structure of the book itself is an experience as important as the plot or any of the characters. Darley ruminates towards the end of *Justine*, wondering if he will have enough time, love and peace of mind to grasp the coherence of the order that lies at the heart of his experiences.[6]

In the following pages, I will read the stratified and complex structure of the novel while bearing in mind some psychoanalytic ideas concerning the structure of the human mind. I will refer to these ideas to highlight the role of the different narrative voices as forming one complex author figure, his mind split and torn, whether between its conscious and unconscious layers or between the different parts of the Self – ego, superego and id.[7] I will focus on the multiple narrative voices and address the conscious intentions of the author in his *prefatory notes*[8] to each of the four volumes, while taking to heart Durrell's own explicit words of caution against the damage too much interpretation can do to the reading experience, if one tries to be too concrete and specific; one has to be as gentle as when one is trying to touch a delicate and rare butterfly.[9]

The Alexandria Quartet: narrative time and narrative voices

The narrative course plotted by Lawrence Durrell in the *Quartet* is a conscious effort to disrupt the prospect of a clear linear plotline that lends itself to simple description.[10] In order to retrace, or even plot, such a linear course, one must review the *Quartet* and put together a narrative continuum. This kind of reading reduces the work to a sum total that constitutes no whole. The work's integrity lies in its fragmentary nature, where the plot has a labyrinthine topography. Durrell created a premeditated fragmentary narrative to highlight the developmental course experienced by the author. The course of writing is in fact a course of development, allowing the author's mind to mature. Having completed the *Quartet*, Durrell noted in an interview that the idea of a work consisting of four volumes is evidence of the maturational process the writer has gone through.[11] The *Quartet*'s plot was put together as a testimony of Durrell's mind and therefore warrants a search for its conscious and unconscious parts. But the author's mind is neither a being nor an entity that lurks between the pages of the book that can be put into simple outlines. It is exactly this facile effort that Durrell's project strives to overcome. The voice and mind of the author are scattered throughout the work as a stream of associations following in each other's footsteps, like memories that surface in one's mind. The plot of the *Quartet* does not validate one theory or another; rather, it is a testimony of the reflective process of the author as he grapples with the existential themes of his life: love, creativity, solitude, alienation and belonging.

According to Durrell, the work's structure rests on three spatial dimensions and one temporal dimension. In his prefatory note to *Balthazar* he wrote that the first three volumes of the *Quartet* are to be treated as siblings and not as sequels to one another. Therefore, he suggests that there is no serial connection between them. They overlap, intermingle and co-exist simultaneously, rather like the three dimensions of space. The only dimension which remains constant is the fourth one, time. But the flow of time is suspended.[12] Durrell therefore asks that we read the first three volumes of the *Quartet* synchronically, without trying to trace them for a linear continuum; rather, he wants us to perceive them as a three-dimensional object in space. The fourth dimension, of time, should be sought, as Durrell proposes, in the fourth volume, which is the only one that can be read as a sequel to the other three volumes.

Durrell uses the flow of time as a psychological event that encompasses the subjective experiences of the protagonists. Riding the crest of the initial success of the *Quartet*, early studies treated Durrell's ambition to base his notion of psychological time on scientific time-space theories as a worthwhile endeavour. John A. Weigel, in his study of Durrell in 1965, wrote that the experiences described in the work seemed to renounce the need to look out there, into the world. In Weigel's opinion, the only real significant sense of time is the individual subjective sense of time. It is only such a subjective sense of time that is a true record of the individual.[13] This overview of the story's chronological continuum is no accident. The romantic tale on which the reader is invited to focus seems to unfurl beyond the groove of time. The reader is initially invited to overlook broader historical aspects of the work, and focus exclusively on the subjective time of the protagonist. Weigel found this to be reflective of the individualistic self-centred outlook of the times. Gerald Goldberg, on the other hand, criticised the emphasis on such romantic notions of the *Quartet* and argued in 1963 that the focus on the subjective time of the protagonist was engaging enough to be considered as the work's focal point only in the first two volumes.[14] He claimed that Durrell's endeavour to make the narrator's subjective experience a nodal point illustrated the weakness of this very axis as the plot unfolds. Reading the first two volumes, it does seem that the tetralogy explores the development of the troubled protagonist, thus claiming its place in the nineteenth-century *Bildungsroman* tradition. As the work unfolds and other voices join in, the author's ironic intention is revealed, placing the subject in a broader context that puts his emotional woes in a very different perspective. Goldberg perceived that as a fundamental flaw. He regarded the prefatory notes seriously and assumed the author had been fully conscious, and in full control of all that was at play in the process of writing. He assumed that the author had been acting as a conscious, coherent and cohesive subject – a notion that I will later challenge. Indeed, if one read the words spoken by Pursewarden to Darley in *Clea* as guidelines, one could see how convincing Durrell's intention could be perceived. Pursewarden urges Darley to write a novel based on its structure analogous with the four winds of heaven, using a common axis to make the whole structure revolve.[15]

The more critical trend towards Durrell's work was gaining momentum in the wake of his later publications, which failed to reap the same acclaim. Herbert Howarth, for example, claimed in 1972 that Durrell's ambition of writing a novel where the individual's destiny was seen to be rightly sacrificed in the interests of the greater collective perhaps reflected his own personal experience but had little to do with the actual reality of Alexandria at that time.[16] Thus, his ambition of writing a meta-structured novel resulted in a hollow plot structure. His lack of any significant connection with the Egyptian population he had written about had turned the structure into a house of cards. Even more scathing reviews addressed Durrell's presumption in using the time and space dimensions as his plot's building blocks. As Steve Franklin noted in 1979, the theory of relativity perhaps served Durrell as an inspiration as implied in the prefatory notes, yet showed no significant innovation in the way it was used. Other critics too found a gap between the expectation

Durrell created and the text itself. Franklin suggested that the reader would do well to skip the prefatory notes and relish the verbal richness and human sensitivity of Durrell's writing.[17]

Such a suggestion to disregard the reflective process of the writer recalls Roland Barthes' call for the reading and interpretation of texts without paying any attention to the figure of the actual writer, as he argued in his seminal work *Death of the Author* (1977). Such a view limits the interpretive perspective on the text, contrary to the hermeneutic view, which reads the text within its overall contexts.[18] According to Hans-Georg Gadamer, the literary text cannot be read in a manner that is alienated and detached of any cultural and biographical element.[19] Franklin argued that Durrell made an unwarranted, artificial, and maybe even gratuitous use of extra-textual theories, like Albert Einstein's (1879–1955) theory of relativity. While this criticism may be relevant, his conclusion, that the text must be read outside any context, seems too far-reaching. Scholars such as Franklin who find the reflective process described in the prefatory notes as irrelevant, misses the point, in my opinion, with their call to regard the author's musings as redundant. I argue, like scholars such as Paul Lorenz, that the actual and biographical voice of Lawrence Durrell, including his explicit preoccupation with certain theories, is as significant a fictional and valid element of the text as are the voices of the protagonists themselves. Lorenz claimed that Lawrence Durrell, as the writer of the work and like its narrator voices, was not an actual figure, but rather a composite of all the voices he had written during his career. By writing the *Quartet*, he assembles himself into a complete, though fragmented and split, character which made sense of his existence through his actions, biography, theories and relationships.[20] David Lowenkron claimed in 1976 that the different narrative voices of the *Quartet* are different representations of the single writer who is 'responsible' for the entire work.[21] In the *meta-novel* genre, narrative voices produce a dialogue within the plot. Each of the narrative voices is seemingly unaware that he is a figment of the author's imagination, and part of a group, and this lack of awareness does not interfere with his seemingly autonomous function as a narrator. Lowenkron ascribed the *Quartet* to this genre, alongside works like André Gide's (1869–1951) *The Counterfeiters*, Doris Lessing's (1919–2013) *The Golden Notebook* and others. The narrative voices are the voices of the author, reflecting his aspiration for recognition as the complex and divided individual he is.

The complexity is further deepened once we take into consideration that even though the structure of the work is deterministic, i.e. determined by the intentions of the writer, there will still be gaps and incoherencies in the text. These can be best looked at by seeking the unconscious undertones of the voices, as suggested by psychoanalytic theory. Thus, the multiple narrative voices' "problem" is no problem and therefore needs no unequivocal solution. It simply adds another dimension to the reading. This is best seen in the fourth volume of the work, *Clea*, which is made of several parts, each with a different narrative voice: Clea's letter to Darley, the diary left by Pursewarden as his will to Darley following his suicide, the account of Darley's return to Alexandria in the wake of the Second World War and others.

This volume does not intend to produce a cohesive narrative thread that connects its different parts. Each part sheds a different light on the plot and on all that was told in the preceding volumes, without venturing to solve the complex questions posed by their labyrinthine plot. The reader is left with open questions even as the work draws to an end.

Though constituting one of the work's strengths, this aspect also poses challenges for the reader who expects the narrative to be conclusive. As Frank Kersnowski wrote in 2010, Durrell seemed to have deliberately built the plot in a manner that disrupts any coherence.[22] Therefore, a conclusion as is expected in a "boy meets girl" type of book is never reached and the reader must grapple with the existential ambiguity that the narrative, and particularly its fourth volume, creates. Even though in many parts, the work reads as if it were a "boy meets girl" kind of novel, the element of surprise as the plot develops and unfurls, disrupts ordinary treatment of such themes. What you thought of as being true, is revealed to be just another layer that you will have to excavate. It is no longer a question of *what the object was that the author attempted to describe*, but rather how *the shadow of the object* was described, or in other words, the impressions left by the author's consciousness.[23] As Pursewarden writes in reference to the function of the artistic endeavour in one's life, when he asks whether the artistic act is simply the white stick with which the blind man finds his way around in the darkness, knowing there is something there but never being able to see it.[24] In conclusion, a contemporary reading of *The Alexandria Quartet* may find earlier reviews of this work, which found it to reflect one scientific theory or another, to be somewhat naïve or even irrelevant. As I will explore in the following pages and as both studies by Michael Haag and Richard Pine of the writing process of the tetralogy show, the whole endeavour by Durrell was to find a cure for his soul, rather than to reflect any scientific or theoretic worldview.[25] The work as a whole stands as testimony to the mind of the author and the existential questions that plagued him during the writing process.

The prefatory notes and the narrative voices

The conscious aspects of the reflective process of the author of the *Quartet* can be seen in the prefatory notes of the four single volumes where he declared his intention. These notes, alongside the workpoints at the end of three of the four volumes, are physically marginal to the text and can almost be overlooked, if one is not careful. However, it is my opinion that they form the framework for the entire work, the fence that encompasses the landscape of this work, the borderlines that mark the mind of the author. No individual consciousness can be encompassed as a single, clear and cohesive essence. Searching for answers in the prefatory notes echoes the proposal made by Gadamer to search for the question that presents itself within the text.[26] The very physical presence of the prefatory notes, surrounding the main body of the work, signifies the clear distinction between the voice of the writer (Lawrence Durrell sitting down to write the *Quartet*) and the various voices of the author (the assembly of the different voices of the narrative) in the work.

Seemingly detached from the plot continuum, the prefatory notes were designed to lay a foundation without which, according to the author, the work as a whole might not be readable.

Despite Durrell's statement that he conceived the *Quartet* years before he had set pen to paper, we can safely assume that in the writing process of each volume, the actual realisation of these plans underwent some changes. It is the writing process, with its intuitive and unconscious elements, that determines the content, rather than the original conscious intention and motivation. Reading the prefatory notes as a continuum permits tracing the different voices of the writer in the reflective process of writing the work. The prefatory notes differ from one another, both in content and in length. Durrell's voice as emanating from them is a biographical and historical voice that seeks to offer a context and backdrop to the fictional voice that follows. This biographical voice is neither more nor less significant than its fictional counterpart, and the two maintain a reciprocal affinity. Durrell's intentions as expressed in these notes are not more valid as a testimony to his reflective process than the main body of text itself. What Durrell chose to reveal in the prefatory notes can be added to what he consciously chose to leave out. Each note features a different aspect of Durrell's voice, which joins the multiplicity of voices in the body of the work. They testify to Durrell's need to prepare the reader for the text itself. He took special pains in his attempt to guide the reader deeper into his state of mind.

The prefatory notes are a direct address to the reader, clarifying, among other things, that in order to understand the text as intended by the writer, a few words of introduction are in place. The main body of the text in itself is not sufficient. A framework is required to present several ideas, a number of rules and some organising principles for readers to use, so they can connect to the text itself. How should one refer to these? Are the prefatory notes a testimony to certain insecurity on the author's part regarding the compelling powers of the text itself? As noted earlier, Durrell had been planning the *Quartet*, or at least its first part, *Justine*, for years before actually writing it. For him, the *Quartet* was the second section in the triptych he had planned as his life work. The first section was *The Black Book* (1938), while the third was *The Avignon Quintet* (1974–1985). The *Quartet*, the pinnacle of his oeuvre, surely in a contemporary perspective, can thus be seen as too important to "abandon" in the hands of the unwitting reader. It is his professed intentions that position him, at least in his own eyes, in the prominent literary status he craved. It may be that the prefatory notes were designed to generate the illusion of continuity and define the author's intention, which is absent from the work itself. Still, they are well worth studying in their own right.

Durrell proposed a sequential reading of the four volumes, which according to him constitute a single work, as well as a word continuum. Every prefatory note, naturally, has its unique historical context, diachronically dovetailing with the respective volume. But there also exists a synchronic link between the prefaces, which I shall try to pinpoint. The prefatory notes as a continuum constitute a meta-structure. I will try to clarify its organising and disorganising principles.

At least four points recur in them. The first point, repeated three times, is the relation between the protagonists and actual living persons. It is a key point, pertaining to the relation between the biographical and fictional elements. The triple denial of any connection between real character and fictional characters underscores the importance of this theme. Can we really take this triple renunciation at face value and accept the author's declarations that the characters in his work are entirely imaginary? That we should not ascribe them any biographical basis? Or should this triple renunciation raise some doubts? I suggest that this triple renunciation can neither succeed nor fail in its mission to put the reader's doubts to rest – rather, it underscores the importance of looking into the relation at play between the work's biographical and fictional elements. Durrell's caution that no such link exists has the opposite effect, prompting readers to address this complex matrix. Furthermore, the phrasing of these words varies from one volume to another, echoing perhaps minute changes in his awareness of the issue. In the first prefatory note to *Justine*, he describes the characters as *invention*. In *Balthazar*, he describes the different persons and situations as *entirely imaginary*, while in *Mountolive*, an almost identical phrasing appears, *purely imaginary*. Durrell's insistence on a stark dichotomous distinction between fiction/imagination and real/living – i.e. between the work's fictional and biographical elements – makes one wonder whether this is an effort to blur the biographical tracks with the fictional details, thus evoking the strong sense of *unheimliche* which is so dominant in the text. it is specifically the confusion between the living and the dead, between the real and the imaginary that alerted Freud's attention when writing about *unheimliche*. It also calls to mind the psychoanalytic defence mechanism of *denial*, designed to cover the tracks left by traumatic mental experiences.

The second recurring point in both *Justine* and *Balthazar* is the city's place in the paradigm of reality versus fiction. In *Justine* he writes that *only the city is real*, while in *Balthazar* he refers to the same city in a manner that is hard to understand at first: *nor could the city be less unreal*. This statement again contains a triple renunciation. The complex, convoluted sentence generates a labyrinthine experience, which the author entices the readers to enter, so that they follow the different narrative levels. For Durrell, the city, both as a metaphor and an actuality, embodies his effort to find an imaginary motherland to replace the homeland he has lost. I will elaborate on the city of Alexandria and its connotations in chapter four.

The third point refers to the structure of the *Quartet*. It is the most complex of all points made in the prefatory notes and appeared in three of them, *Balthazar*, *Mountolive* and *Clea*. Durrell dwells on it considerably. It is first cited in the statement that the *Quartet*'s volumes constitute *a group*. At this point the author makes no mention of the number of the volumes which will follow in due course, or the relations between them. According to Michael Haag, work on the *Quartet*'s first volume, *Justine*, took longer than the other volumes.[27] The last three volumes were completed in less than two years, between 1958 and 1959, while the first volume kept Durrell busy for roughly five years. Its writing began in 1952 but it was not until 1957 that he completed it, having moved to the south of France with his third wife, Claude-Marie Forde (née Vincendon), known mostly as Claude, (1925–1967). While writing *Justine*, as evident in his letters from that period, Durrell was far from certain that he could complete this ambitious project. In *Balthazar*, written after the conceptual framework for the entire tetralogy was clear in his mind, Durrell defined the kinship relations between its volumes. Evidently, by now he had a better idea of the project's scope and what had been so far a mere group became a family. The second and third volumes created siblings to the first book, while the fourth volume formed a sequel. This prefatory note is the *raison d'être* of the entire work. Durrell notes that the structure at hand comprises four parts and is movable rather than static. He refers to it as a four-decker novel. The word *decker* denotes a level. It is therefore a structure that comprises several layers. He ushers readers into a complex reading experience, promising a journey into a symbolic, hierarchic mystery labyrinth.

The fourth point appears in *Balthazar*, where the intentions of the author are presented in the most detailed and elaborate manner. Durrell takes the reader on a journey through a multidisciplinary field of modern science and literature alike. He voices his despair with the conventional literary structure, repeated also in the prefatory note to *Clea*. He turns to Einstein's theory of relativity in an effort to find new paradigms to express his literary ideas. He suggests that the literary form he has created in the *Quartet* represents the theory of relativity, just as the writings of Proust and Joyce represent the theories of time by the French philosopher Henri Bergson (1895–1941). Durrell was in thrall to Einstein's discovery that the perception of space was bound together with the perception of time in the universe in a non-linear relationship. The relative unfolding of time as an organising principle allowed Durrell to abandon both the traditional novel structure and the idea of objective truth. Durrell declares that the story he tells aims to interweave objective and subjective views of reality. Such a matrix will result, for example, in the same characters making different appearances in different geographical and cultural contexts. Thus they will disrupt any uniform, cohesive perception of them or of the meanings of their actions. At the end of the day, no objective judgement could be passed on the moral stance and actions of the protagonists. They will be perceived in their full spectrum of appearances, while their actions and relationships will acquire unstable and varying meanings due to the organising principle of relativity. Durrell emphasises in *Clea* that, since time is relative and multidirectional, it is impossible to reach a total conclusion of the plot's chain of events. He declares that the *Quartet*'s plot may theoretically stretch ad infinitum, or at least so long as he is willing to pursue the word continuum that he has started. In a way, Durrell remains true to this proclamation, as some of the characters portrayed in the *Quartet* indeed feature in later works, like *The Avignon Quintet*.

Durrell asks the reader to treat the *Quartet* as a living entity that outlasts the actual act of reading. By the end of each of the four volumes, an additional part appears that also seems external to the continuum of the book itself. This part is referred to by Durrell as *workpoints*. These are an assortment of remarks by the *Quartet*'s protagonists, poems by Durrell and other poets and his reflections on events in the plot. In *Clea*, Durrell writes that these workpoints show the reader the many opportunities still left to explore in the *Quartet*, even as the reader has reached the end. These are the author's attempt to stall the *Quartet*'s demise (the physical conclusion of the reading experience). As the *Quartet* has at its heart the relativity of time and hence the relativity of truth and our relative understanding of its voices, the workpoints allow future readers to draw their own different sequels for the entire work. By concluding three volumes of the *Quartet* with these workpoints, the author performs two significant acts.[28] First, he defies his own authority as the author. Each reader is welcome to follow the *Quartet* according to the clues provided by Durrell in the workpoints. The reader is invited to become the author of the text and join the extensive pantheon of narrator voices. This invitation chimes with the relativity spirit. The imagination of the reader is invoked and he is invited to make the *Quartet* his own. The second act is the renunciation of an end to the *Quartet*, that is, the renunciation of death. The *Quartet* does not end, nor can it end, just like time itself, according to the theory of relativity. Durrell espouses Einstein's theory as it helps him sustain the *destruction of history* experience, described at length in chapter four. When time does not end, but is rather sustained in a cyclic periodicity where each cycle unearths another level of the stratified, infinite plot structure, the story continues forever.

Durrell acknowledges the grandiosity of his ambitions and accepts that this attempt may consign him to the margins of literature, as unfortunately indeed happened eventually. He also admits that he is of course not the first twentieth-century author to use these means. His attempt to create a plot with a structure that outlives chronological time, a plot with an end point that may also be the starting point of resumed reading, gained recognition and esteem in the 1960s, and inspired several writers. For example, one of the emerging South American writers in the Western culture of that decade, part of the Latin American Boom, was the exiled Belgian-Argentinian author Julio Cortázar, who employed a similar technique when writing his major prose work, *Hopscotch*, published in 1963.[29] As Bloom writes in his analysis of the work of Cortázar, his use of a literary structure that does not follow linear time but rather an associative continuum stands as a tribute to the writing of Lawrence Durrell.[30]

The structure of *The Alexandria Quartet*

The topographical view of the mind, i.e. the mind as a place, is one of the basic tenets of psychoanalytical thinking, deeply bound up with the concepts of belonging and attachment. Freud's conviction regarding the dominance of *the unconscious* in determining human behaviour is a topographical argument that sees the human mind as divided.[31] As this is not a psychoanalytic textbook, I shall not elaborate on psychoanalytic theory beyond what is strictly necessary. As I have explained in the previous chapters, psychoanalytic theory is not used in this study as an objective methodological instrument to analyse Durrell's work, but rather as an inspiration to deepen its interpretation. Generally speaking, Freud proposed two topographical models. The first differentiates three mental systems: the unconscious, the preconscious and the conscious. The second model differentiates between the three parts of the Self: ego, superego and id. Each such system is marked by a different process and content. The first topographic model conceptualised by Freud makes its first major appearance in the seventh chapter of his book on the interpretation of dreams.[32] In this chapter, Freud began to develop his theories on the structure, dynamics and contents of the unconscious, based on the analysis of dreams (mainly his own but also of his early patients and colleagues). He suggested that the essence of the contents of the unconscious is the product of repression of conflictual ideas. These ideas are repressed to protect the mind of the individual from unwarranted conflicts between what he desires and what he deems to be unacceptable. Freud suggested that the unconscious contents relentlessly strive to emerge into the awareness of the individual one way or another. That is the *dynamic* nature of the mind. Yet the unconscious was not described by Freud as a mere storeroom for repressed and forbidden sexual contents that sought to gain entrance to awareness through *dreams*, *symptoms* and *slips of the tongue*. He also believed that it was in the unconscious that the creativity of the individual evolved and matured. It was in the unconscious level of the psyche that the most creative thoughts were conceived, the place where artistic and literary works were hatched. Freud went so far as to say that it was the poet who was first to arrive at the deepest and most original ideas, well before the psychoanalyst.[33]

There are three main layers that I wish to emphasis in the structure of the *Quartet*. The first layer belongs to the narrative voices, the second layer is the complex relationships described throughout the book, and the third layer is the political reality of 1930s–1940s Egypt.[34] These layers maintain different topographic relations in each volume of the work. Often they are "superimposed," hiding one another, with one layer serving as a *screen memory* for another, deeper layer. For example, in the first two volumes, *Justine* and *Balthazar*, the plot has its almost exclusive focus on the romantic relations between the protagonists (the second layer), with only very subtle insinuations concerning external events. It is this gentle insinuation that sets the stage for that which will only come to light in the third volume – the political reality which assumes great significance for understanding the protagonists' relationships (the second layer) in the previous volume. It seems to render the focus on the reflective aspects of the narrative (the first layer) as superfluous and meaningless. It is only in the last volume that an attempt is made to weave together the three layers, or in other words: an attempt to make the unconscious conscious.

The topography created by Durrell is a metaphoric container that he planned to fill with personal experiences of his complex sense of belonging. The entire work is a vessel wherein the author seeks to locate himself. Durrell places the "important" contents that serve as the driving force of the entire work in the unconscious level, which is then gradually and masterfully revealed to the reader. This multi-layered topography is Durrell's attempt at returning to a place from which he had been exiled. As a multi-layered place, it is forever *unheimliche*, both homely and strange; surprising the reader time and again with the new discoveries it yields. What seems at one moment to stand at the heart of the work, like his affairs, trysts etc., is later dented and virtually overshadowed by the latest discovery. What was familiar and homely, *heimliche*, become threatening and deadly *unheimliche*. The topography of the story becomes unsettling, offering no stable ground. Nothing remains familiar or predictable. The author feels like a stranger within his own consciousness. His actual wanderings and writing made him look for a place where he could re-constitute his sense of belonging. The place where he finds himself offers no stable and secure attachment but mirrors the treacherous realities formed by his choices and the interpersonal relations he has established during his life.

The three layers of the plot

The first layer is dense with several narrative voices, some of which also appear as protagonists, telling the story from a particular perspective. This layer constitutes the conscious continuum of the narrator, the conscious layer of the work's topographical structure. The narrative voices and reflective continuum form a constant feature of the entire work, like a recurring rhyme in the turbulent music of the *Quartet*. This layer belongs to Darley, the conscious voice of the narrative, whose stay on the island is described as an exile from the moment he arrives there with the daughter of his dead lover, Melissa. While on the island he writes his memories from his stay in Alexandria. It is the *elusive memory*.[35] His voice dominates this layer, which is laden with philosophical and psychological reflections on love, relationships, writing, literature and death – the key themes in all the books of Lawrence Durrell. The reading experience is as of a diary or the conversation of the patient in therapy. It calls for identification with the narrative voice. It is the only one heard. It is an autobiographical voice filled with the experiences as a survivor of a protracted exile and loss marked by fierce emotions. Darley employs the first person voice, addressing no one in particular, in a clear, consistent manner. He speaks like a lonely man who has lost his sense of belonging and knows not whom he addresses when he talks. His voice echoes in a vacuum, reflecting experiences of modern despair and alienation from which he strives to escape.

The second layer describes the relationships between the different protagonists of the *Quartet*. It constitutes the preconscious of the work's topographic structure, where Durrell attempts to rescue Darley from his solitary and singular narration of the story. Although Darley remains dominant, Durrell brings in other narrative voices, expanding the horizon of the story. The perception of reality that underpins this layer is polyphonic. Durrell employs several literary forms to usher in different voices, mainly using excerpts from letters and notes addressed to Darley. The polyphony of voices emanates from somewhere deeper, its existence hitherto only insinuated. The truth laid out in the first layer transpires as just one version of reality. Other voices offer different versions of the same story, casting doubt on the original version. Darley, the main narrative voice, the conscious aspect of the story, is no longer the singular focal point of the story. His voice is counterbalanced and contextualised by the other narrative, preconscious voices, whose stories are as valid and relevant as his own. The singular turns plural.

The third layer is the turbulent and dark political reality in the pre–Second World War years in Europe and the Middle East. It lays down the unconscious ground of the topographic structure. This layer illuminates the events of the plot as driven by deep, underlying social and political forces, while the personal-subjective experiences portrayed are depicted as derivatives and symptomatic of these political forces. This layer lurks like a shadow that makes the occasional appearance as an insinuation in the first two volumes of the plot, emerging in the third volume. Having been revealed to the reader, it irrevocably changes the way the work is read, understood and interpreted. All the preceding events have their meaning altered and are seen in a new light. Their former meaning seems irrelevant, anachronistic, a vestige of a premature, monotonous worldview. Durrell employs this layer for telling "the truth." It is the unearthing of this layer that seems to lend the work its depth and full scope. While the first layer reflected the voice of the subjective individual, with the second layer reflecting the voices of relationships, the third layer completes the picture, providing the wider perspective for the two previous layers. As well as being the underground, unconscious driving force behind the subjective thoughts and relationships described in the book, it also constitutes a framework. It is the outer boundary that frames the landscape of the entire tale.

The three layers are contained within the boundaries of the entire story, the prefatory notes and the workpoints, as the skin of the individual holds within him the various parts of his body and mind. They are relative to each other in a non-linear, steady fashion, and do not point to any straightforward developmental process. The three layers circle in and around each other. Durrell gradually exposes the reader to the way in which the three interrelate. As reading commences, one gets the impression that the tetralogy only concerns the subjective tormented experience of the protagonist. Later, however, alongside this vein, the reader is also exposed to the role of others in his life. Only then is the third layer introduced, encompassing the entire tale. It changes the perspective, i.e. the location, of the voice of the individual and his specific gravity relative to his surroundings. The body of the story is a complex self, containing within it diverse and even contradictory elements, held together by the skin of a single purpose – seeking a place that will contain the quest for a sense of belonging, a sense of homeland where the individual can feel at home within himself.

The entire tale, and particularly its portrayal of Alexandria, as will be discussed in chapter four, stands as testimony to the self of the writer and his effort to find an imaginary homeland experience to make up for the loss, or total absence, of an actual homeland.

The voices of the narrative

The voyage towards home is told by a choir of narrative voices. The narrator of the tetralogy is a multifaceted character. His plural identity rather than a singular voice is pivotal to this work. This characterisation of a non-uniform self that hold together different, complementary and contradictory voices, is inspired by psychoanalytical works by Freud, Otto Rank, Georg Groddeck and the philosopher Francis John Mott (1901–1980). Early on in the *Quartet* Justine teases Darley and says that if *she* was the writer of the tale, she would use a voice of many dimensions, showing the full range of colours available in the portrayal of all the possible views of reality.[36] It is indeed exactly that that Durrell in fact does in the story. The multi-dimensional narrative voice reflects the psychoanalytic notion of the multifaceted nature of the self, the split self. Similar to the jigsaw-like plot he created to establish the complex structure of the story, Durrell accordingly put together the voices of the narrative.

Studies of the *Quartet* have often raised the question of who the narrator was in *The Alexandria Quartet*. This question can also assume a different form: how many narrative voices are there in *The Alexandria Quartet?* I argue that the multiplicity of narrative voices reflects Durrell's efforts to show that the individual has no single, sovereign voice, but rather a multitude of voices. This multiplicity produces a non-cohesive identity that does not easily lend itself to definitions, if at all. It is the contradictions and tensions generated among the different narrative voices that produce the rich, diverse and challenging tapestry of the novel.

The most dominant narrative voice is Darley, the narrator and author of the *Quartet*'s first volume, *Justine*. Darley's manuscript of *Justine* forms the basis for the following volumes. It is the purported original, primeval text, which also features other narrative voices. For example, it quotes at length from a novel by Arnauti, Justine's first husband. Darley himself quotes at length from the diaries of Justine, thereby designating her as a narrative voice, on top of her position as a protagonist in the novel. Nor is it just Justine's diaries that Darley reads. Excerpts from the diaries written by her husband, Nessim Hosnani, also form part of *Justine*'s narrative, casting him in a similar position, as a protagonist in the story and a narrative voice alternately. Another major narrative voice belongs to Dr. Balthazar, Darley's friend, who reads Darley's manuscript of *Justine*, and comments upon it through a manuscript of his own, called *the interlinear*. The volume that Balthazar reads is the same one available to the real readers of the *Quartet*, us. This act of reading seems to cast Balthazar as one of the real readers of the story, but also as a narrative voice, which gives him power over the development of the tetralogy. The voice and figure of Balthazar transcend the lines of biography and fiction and wander to and fro between these two realms. He is at once an actual and fictional voice. The reading of Balthazar is not passive. Having read the manuscript, he adds significant notes that test Darley's perception of reality, showing him his errors. His narrative voice, through his notes which form the core of the *Quartet*'s second volume bearing his name, is the conscious gate that allows the work's unconscious parts to burst forth into the narrative.

Another narrative voice that appears later in the novel and affects its course is Pursewarden, whom Lawrence Durrell marked as his double, alter-ego and at times superego. In a 1960 interview, Durrell confirmed that Darley and Pursewarden constituted the two dominant aspects of the voice of the author.[37] Pursewarden shares some biographical details with Darley, but he is a more mature version of the latter. On top of working for the British administration in Alexandria (as Lawrence Durrell did himself), he is an author of world renown, which Darley can only hope for at this early stage of his career. Pursewarden has many connections in Alexandria with businessmen and intellectuals, and is naturally an attraction for many women lured by his spells. Pursewarden is everything that the sensitive, insecure Darley will not let himself be at this stage. His letters and extensive parts from his diaries, including his suicide letter he addresses to Darley, take up a considerable portion of the fourth volume of the novel.

The third volume, *Mountolive*, is delivered exclusively by a narrative voice of undisclosed identity. Darley, the main narrative voice of the other three volumes, appears there as a fairly marginal character. The story of this volume constitutes the "objective" dimension of the multi-layered structure created by Durrell. David Mountolive is a British diplomat in Egypt and this volume recounts his experiences in the years leading up to the Second World War, beginning at an earlier point in time than *Justine* did. This volume sees the third layer of the plot, the political reality, surfacing time and again. It is here that Mountolive finds out that Nessim and Justine Hosnani are involved in a Coptic scheme to smuggle arms to the Jewish underground in British Mandate Palestine, with the purpose of thwarting the burgeoning Muslim forces in Egypt. All the characters from the other volumes feature in this volume, though in a perspective altogether different, which underplays, for example, the complex dimension of their mutual affairs. Accordingly, rather than as an authentic reflection of her, Justine's romantic escapades emerge as schemes designed to dazzle Darley, Pursewarden and other men, lest they disclose the political plot hatched by her and Nessim. Moreover, the narrator's reflections, dominant in the first two volumes, have no presence in this volume. All the misgivings and alienation that preoccupied the narrative voices in the first two volumes, marking them out as part of a *Bildungsroman*, can no longer be found in this volume, which represents the ultimate *raison d'être* of the work itself – humans, with their personal vacillations and misgivings, are but pawns in the hands of greater, inexplicable powers.

The fourth volume, *Clea*, is a symposium of several narrative voices. The voice of Clea, the third major female protagonist of the tetralogy, becomes central with the letter she addresses to Darley, where she unfolds her version of the events described in *Justine*. Pursewarden's suicide letter, addressed to Darley, becomes another dominant theme. Pursewarden, Darley's *Doppelgänger*, takes his own life worried as he is about his failure, in his capacity as an employee of the British administration, to uncover Nessim and Justine's political scheme.[38] His letter stands as personal will and a guide for the perplexed Darley. The fourth volume relates Darley's return to the city. He can no longer use his personal woes to support the full weight of the plot with its existential implications. This is no longer about the personal fate of one individual or another; it is about the adversities of an entire community. It is no longer the fate of Darley's lover or his personal fulfilment as a writer that is at stake, but rather the fate of Egyptian society at large, and later the fate of the Jewish settlement in Palestine.

The multiple narrative voices do not pose the identity of the narrator as a logical puzzle to solve, but rather as a testimony of Lawrence Durrell's *Weltanschauung* that acknowledges the dominance of the fragmented and unsettling unconscious elements in the human psyche. They allow him to assemble the novel, with its diverse narrative voices, as a finely woven matrix. A crude cut of any of the threads will leave them lifeless. Therefore my analysis in the next sections of this study offers a scrupulous yet careful diachronic attention and interpretation of two aspects of the narrative voices, so as to bring out some themes that lie hidden within their folds while leaving their beauty unharmed.

The narrator as a wounded hero

Reading the first words uttered by the narrative voice is akin in my mind to listening to the words first spoken by the patient. It is the beginning, the beginning of the story, the beginning of the life about to be shared and explored. The first words in the *Quartet* are spoken by Darley, without naming him just yet. Following an exposition of the landscape and engulfing stormy weather he writes that he has escaped to the island, carrying with him some books and a child whose mother is Melissa.[39] The first act that Durrell attributes to the protagonist, who is also a narrative voice, is the act of escape. The reader has yet to find out what it is that he escaped from or where exactly he has arrived. The books are first on his list of objects he has taken along, closely followed by the child. We have yet to know which books, but their position on top of the list shows Darley's priorities. Books, and perhaps the tradition they stand for, come before the child, for whom he is probably responsible. They are portrayed as his companions. He continues with an expression of self-doubt and is baffled at his own choice of the word *escape* to describe his way of arrival. He thereby introduces himself as *an anti-hero*, unsure of his motivations. As early as this stage we realise there is another, yet to be identified, element that seems to govern his actions and their representation in his writing. Durrell introduces this narrative voice as possessing a split mind. As of this point, his reflective process will form one of the focal points of the entire work. The narrator is not there merely to recount the tale, but also to lay bare his reflections regarding the events he recounts. But his conscious voice, a manifestation of his ego, points to another region in his mind, where additional knowledge seems to lurk.

The storm described by Darley in the opening paragraph represents his own turbulent mental state. He does not know yet what has brought him to the island, but he can see that the local residents think of him as sick if he chose to come to the remote island to recover and heal himself. Several paragraphs later, he reveals that his sickness is in the most intimate and private part of his being. He, like all people he imagines to surround him, suffers a wounded sexuality. He is left bruised by his sexual and romantic affairs in Alexandria. As early as the opening, Durrell marks its end and his conclusion regarding the consequences and repercussions of giving in to *modern love*: the protagonist is sexually wounded, retreating to heal in seclusion. Darley addresses the readers directly and thereby sets in motion the dialogue-in-writing that he invites them to embark upon. Despite his apparent solitude on the island, he is not alone – he talks to the local villagers and writes his testimony. He invites the reader to witness the goings-on around him. Darley is preoccupied with his memories from the city he escaped, Alexandria, and the friends he left behind, Justine, Melissa (who had died since), Nessim and Balthazar. These four characters are his first port of call as he tries to trace back the chain of events that led him to the island. The hand that pulls the strings of the story seems to be fate, or the city of Alexandria, the focus of this entire tale, as specified in chapter four.

The opening scene sees Lawrence Durrell cast the narrative voice in a situation of mythological proportions: a lone or virtually lone hero, on a remote island, far away from anywhere familiar. He is in exile, engulfed by memories of the place from which he has arrived. He has an experience of injury to contend with, physical and mental. He tries to overcome this wound so as to return to the place where it all began. He has a child in his care who is not his offspring, a reminder of his dead lover, and he also has his books as companions. For him, these books stand for his past; marking him out as a member of the culture and tradition he came from, while the child constitutes a faint promise of the future to come. He faces the elements as his memories keep crowding him in a process of reconstructing his past. He waits, contemplating the ruins of his life, recalling *the old man* of Alexandria who had suffered a similar fate.[40] Durrell's approach to this mythological scene, where a hero faces the elements of his fate, begs the question: who is the hero that Durrell has in mind, the inspiration for this important scene?

The clue appears a few lines later when he refers to Mark Antony (82–30 BC), the Roman general and politician, whose life history is recounted by Plutarch, in his classic *The Life of Antony*.[41] Durrell refers to the time that saw Antony strike a political pact with Cleopatra, queen of Egypt, which turns into a pact of love. One of the climaxes of this pact came three years prior to Antony's death, when he divided the assets of the Empire between the couple's mutual offspring and set out on a glorious triumph through the streets of Alexandria. This manifestation of the pact, which made Antony abandon Rome and leave behind disgruntled and betrayed allies and his wife and children, caused a grave rift in the Roman Empire, which actually marked the beginning of its demise. Antony's former companions declared war on Cleopatra. Antony remained loyal to her. Following the marine battle of Actium, the two returned to Alexandria defeated, where Antony met his end. The circumstances of his death have several versions. One version suggests that he killed himself, having wrongly assumed that Cleopatra had taken her own life before him. Another version has him murdered by an Egyptian military. By the end of *Justine*, Durrell quotes Cavafy's 1911 poem *The God Abandons Antony*.[42] It is no coincidence. Like Antony, Darley pays a heavy price for his romantic choice. Durrell draws a threefold synchronic nexus between Darley, who lives on an island having been forced to leave Alexandria, Mark Antony, who put the Roman Empire in danger for his Alexandrian love interest, and the Egyptian-Greek poet, Constantine P. Cavafy (1863–1933). The price of love, according to Durrell, is being abandoned as experienced by Cavafy's

Antony. Durrell employs Cavafy's original text as a multi-dimensional interpretation: it helps him constitute the myth of Antony the hero, who sacrifices all for his love, causing havoc as a result.[43] It is through the figure of Antony that he expresses his *raison d'être*. As it later transpires, the "sacrifice" made by Darley was in vain. As the plot unfolds, the woman he thought was his lover, for whom he sacrificed so much (Justine), is portrayed as a schemer, who has seduced him so as to promote the clandestine plot to smuggle arms to Palestine. But the "truth" about Justine is yet to unfold for Darley at this point. It is only in *Balthazar* that he finds out, with the visit of another narrative voice, Dr. Balthazar, as another layer of the "truth" comes to light.

The narrator as critical commentator

Two additional narrative voices appear in the second volume, *Balthazar*, and join Darley, the dominant voice in the *Quartet*'s first volume. Like Darley himself, these voices serve both as narrators, making textual contributions to this work and as protagonists who form part of its plot. This dual presence recurs and reinforces the stratified nature of the work, underscoring the complexity of the fictional narrative voice. These narrative voices represent critical voices that treat Darley's version of the truth as immature and naïve, shackled still by the romantic notion of love. Their mission is to show him the truth and help him regain his sense of stability in life. Their intervention in the plot is that of caring, responsible but formidable parents who fear for the welfare of their child and seek to right his follies with love and discipline. They sound the voice of reality, the responsible adults and representatives of the superego, trying to help Darley adjust to reality and deal with the demands of the real world from which he has escaped.

The first parental voice to represent the critical superego aspect is Pursewarden, a British diplomat serving as cultural attaché of the British administration in Egypt and a renowned writer and poet. The second voice is that of Dr. Balthazar, Egyptian physician of French descent, who resides in Alexandria and dabbles in additional pursuits, like chairing a secret Kabballah study group and other esoteric scriptures. Each of them writes to Darley to reproach him for his futile pursuit of love. Pursewarden writes that Darley's wish to rewrite reality to fit his narcissist needs and vindicate his infatuations is understandable, but constitutes an illusion that must be dispelled in due course, so as not to endanger himself and his friends. Pursewarden's statement is a criticism levelled at the ego as represented by Darley. While Darley applies himself to wish-fulfilment through his relationships with women around him, spurred on by sexual drives masked as romantic passions, Pursewarden argues that following his wishes is a futile and even dangerous act, as the fate of man is determined by greater powers. The self does not actually exist as a cohesive framework, but fashions its activities as reactions to the people surrounding it. Any external change, whether real or imagined, will bring about an adjustment in the position of the self.

The second parental voice, Balthazar, is equally scathing when addressing Darley, chastising him for his attitude. His words are rife with irony and cynicism. His tone is that of a concerned but harsh parent, alert to the mischiefs of his son. He reproaches him for believing he could find truth in his own reflective process. He tears into him, saying that truth is never written or manifest. He implores Darley to question the validity and sincerity of his account (*Justine*) and search elsewhere for the truth (*the interlinear*). According to him, Darley's own words should be the last place to look for the truth. Truth, he contends, is never fully reflected in one's own account. Balthazar's declarations contradict Darley's best efforts. He sees no point in the self-expression and reflective process that Darley applies himself to. He won't find truth this way. The writing process itself is described by Balthazar as a process of deceit. The written material, according to him, has no truth to it – no one is ever going to pour their heart out on paper, not just because of the limitations of art, but also because of the fear of uttering the truth. Balthazar stands for the censorious part of the superego, which will not allow the self free rein and even fears lest its utterance proves harmful. He perceives the efforts of the ego to find self-expression, like Darley's endeavours, naïve at best and even destructive.

I suggest reading these conflicts between Darley, Pursewarden and Balthazar in the light of the relentless battle as waged between the ego, which strives to assert and fulfil its wishes, and the superego, which reins in the ego's drive so as to regulate and protect it from itself and from the chains imposed by reality. This conflictual process continues throughout the life of the individual and is resolved or mitigated, through a creative sublimation of one's urges, or by developing pathological emotional and mental symptoms. Durrell offers something other than a sublimated end to this particular conflictual instance. In the *Quartet*, the narrative voices representing the superego lose their grip. Pursewarden kills himself, having realised he misjudged Nessim and Justine's involvement in the scheme to smuggle arms to Palestine. Balthazar lives on but no longer has the same formidable influence upon him. Darley, representing the ego, is left alone, free to do as he wishes, without the protection and restriction of the superego. Being left alone will allow him to give in to those parts in his psyche that Balthazar and Pursewarden have tried to warn him against – the uninhibited parts that only seek unmitigated pleasure and pursuit of desires. In other words, the removal of the critical voices will allow his sexuality to express itself, as will be demonstrated in chapter four. The death and therefore absence of the superego allows the surfacing of unconscious materials that may compromise the cohesion of the self. The protagonist is left with no protection from his worst enemy, himself, or to be more precise, from the unconscious parts of his psyche that seek expression at all cost, even at the price of injuring Darley himself.

Notes

1 Durrell, Lawrence, 1957a, *Justine*, London: Faber & Faber, p. 77.
2 Eskin, Stanley, 1962, "Durrell's Themes in the *Alexandria Quartet*", *Texas Quarterly*:43–60.
3 Boccia, Micahel, 1989, "Lawrence Durrell's *Alexandria Quartet*: Novel and Palimpsest", in *Form as Content and Rhetoric in the Modern Novel*, New York: Peter Lang, pp. 149–181.
4 Bork, Alfred, 1963, "Durrell and Relativity", *The Centennial Review*, 16:191–203.

5 Whitman, Aldan, 1970, "Durrell in Despair of Future of Man", *New York Times*, March 20, p. 14.
6 Durrell, Lawrence, 1957a, *Justine*, London: Faber & Faber, p. 221.
7 The scope and intention of this study do not allow a thorough study of these ideas except as they are relevant to the interpretation of the *Quartet*. For further reading, I suggest starting with Jean Laplanche and Jean-Bertrand Pontalis' excellent study of all major psychoanalytic concepts, interpreted through modern critical lens, *The Language of Psychoanalysis*, published by Karnac Books in 1973. Also, Jean-Michel Quinodoz's *Reading Freud* is an excellent way of getting acquainted with Freud's writings.
8 This is the term Durrell himself uses, in *Clea*, for the author's notes of the books. They appear in three of the four single volumes of the *Quartet* only when they were first published individually, but were mostly omitted in the single volume which was first published in 1962.
9 Durrell, Lawrence, 1980b, *A Smile in the Mind's Eye*, New York: Universe Books, p. 18.
10 One secondary evidence of Durrell's wish to blur the linear chronological account can be found in his habit of omitting dates in his correspondence. This habit made it extremely difficult for his biographers to put his multiple correspondences in chronological order and attracted ample reproach from his addressees, including T. S. Eliot.
11 Young, Kenneth, 1959, "A Dialogue with Durrell", *Encounter*, 1/6:62. As I will discuss in the final chapter, it is debatable whether Durrell originally intended to write a four-volume book or whether the three volumes after *Justine* were written as he realised that *Justine* on its own did not suffice. The issue is discussed at length by Michael Haag, a strong advocate of the latter opinion. It seems that Durrell himself was not too clear on this. The point remains unresolved. Haag, Michael, 2012b, "The *Alexandria Quartet*- from One Volume to Four", *Deus Loci*, 13:64–74.
12 Durrell, Lawrence, 1958a, *Balthazar*, London: Faber & Faber, p. 9.
13 Weigel, John A., 1965, *Lawrence Durrell*, New York: Twayne Publishers Inc., p. 85.
14 Goldberg, Gerald, 1963, "The Search for the Artist in Some Recent British Fiction", *South Atlantic Quarterly*, 62:387–401.
15 Durrell, Lawrence, 1960, *Clea*, London: Faber & Faber, p. 135.
16 Howarth, Herbert, 1972, "Durrell Snapped in a Library", *London Magazine*, 12:71–84.
17 Franklin, Steve, 1979, "Space-Time and Creativity in Lawrence Durrell's the *Alexandria Quartet*", *Perspectives on Modern Literature*, 5:55–61.
18 Barthes, Roland, 1977, "Death of the Author", in *Image, Music, Text*, trans. Heath Stephen, London: Fontana Press.
19 Gadamer, Hans Georg, 2004, *Truth and Method*, 2nd Edition, New York: Continuum Press.
20 Lorenz, Paul, "Who Is This Larry Durrell Character After All", *Thalia*, 15:24–31.
21 Lowenkron, David, 1976, "The Metanovel", *College English*, 38:345–355.
22 Kersnowski, Frank, 2010, "The *Alexandria Quartet*: A Reconsideration", *Sewanee Review*, 118/3:381–392.
23 The term "The Shadow of the Object" was originally used by Freud in his "Mourning and Melancholy" essay where he described the effects of a loss upon the mind of the individual. Freud claimed that the sadness, and in worse cases the depression, experienced by mourners is evident of the way the memory of the lost person (the shadow) fell upon the mind of the individual. Freud, Sigmund, 1915, "Mourning and Melancholy", in J. Strachey, ed., *The Standard Edition of the Complete Psychological Works of Sigmund Freud*, trans. J. Strachey, Vol. XIV, London: Hogarth Press, pp. 237–258. This term was later explored by Bollas. Bollas, Christopher, 1987, *The Shadow of the Object: Psychoanalysis of the Unthought Known*, London: Free Association Books.
24 Durrell, Lawrence, 1960, *Clea*, London: Faber & Faber, p. 134.
25 Haag, Michael, 2004, *Alexandria, City of Memory*, London: Yale University Press, pp. 318–330; Pine, Richard, 2005, *Lawrence Durrell: The Mindscape*, Corfu: Durrell School of Corfu.
26 Gadamer, Hans Georg, 2004, *Truth and Method*, 2nd Edition, New York: Continuum Press, p. 22.

27 Haag, Michael, 2004, *Alexandria, City of Memory*, London:Yale University Press.
28 Mountolive is the only volume that has no workpoints, as it is the one volume which is not narrated by Darley, Durrell's main protagonist and narrative voice.
29 Colas, Santiago, 2005, "Inventing Autonomies, Meditations on Julio Cortázar and the Politics of Our Time", *The New Centennial Review*, 5/2:1–34.
30 Bloom, Harold, 2005, *Julio Cortázar*, Philadelphia: Chelsea House Publications, pp. 87–90. Bloom actually traces this influence back to Durrell, rather than to other writers who employed a similar technique. He offers an anecdote and reveals that it was Carol Dunlop (1946–1982), Cortázar's third wife, who translated The *Alexandria Quartet* into Spanish at the time when Cortázar was writing *Hopscotch*.
31 Freud, Sigmund, 1912c, "A Note on the Unconscious in Psycho-Analysis", in J. Strachey, ed., *The Standard Edition of the Complete Psychological Works of Sigmund Freud*, trans. J. Strachey, Vol. VIII, London: Hogarth Press, pp. 433–435.
32 Freud, Sigmund, 1900, "Interpretation of Dreams", in J. Strachey, ed., *The Standard Edition of the Complete Psychological Works of Sigmund Freud*, trans. J. Strachey, Vol. IV & V, London: Hogarth Press.
33 Freud, Sigmund, 1908, "Creative Writers and Day-Dreaming", in J. Strachey, ed., *The Standard Edition of the Complete Psychological Works of Sigmund Freud*, trans. J. Strachey, Vol. IX, London: Hogarth Press, pp. 141–154.
34 For further reading of the political situation in Alexandria, see Diboll, Mike, 2004, *Lawrence Durrell's Alexandria Quartet in Its Egyptian Context*, London: Edwin Mellen Press Ltd.
35 Kristeva, Julia, 1991, *Strangers to Ourselves*, trans. L. S. Roudiez, New York: Columbia University Press, p. 23.
36 Durrell, Lawrence, 1957a, *Justine*, London: Faber & Faber, p. 27.
37 Ingersoll, Earl G., 1998, *Lawrence Durrell: Conversations*, London: Associated University Press, p. 63.
38 Pursewarden's suicide has a personal angle to it as well. Throughout the *Quartet* it is hinted that he has been having an illicit sexual relationship with his sister Lisa since their childhood. Mountolive's return to Alexandria spells the end of this affair, causing him great anguish.
39 Durrell, Lawrence, 1957a, *Justine*, London: Faber & Faber, p. 13.
40 Durrell identifies the old man as the poet C. P. Cavafy.
41 Plutarch, 1958, *Lives of the Noble Grecians and Romans*, New York: Bennet and Klopfer, pp. 1110–1153.
42 Cavafy, C. P., 1992, *Collected Poems*, ed., George Savidis, Trans. Edmund Keeley and Philip Sherrard, Revised Edition, Princeton, NJ: Princeton University Press, p. 27.
43 Hirst, Anthony, 2004, "The Old Poet of the City: Cavafy in Darley's Alexandria", in Lawrence Durrell and the Greek World, London: Associated University Press, pp. 106–120.

3

DREAMS AND DREAMING

The four volumes of the *Quartet* are replete with references to dreams, whether in the form of accounts or in the use of the word *dream*. The English *dream* and German *träumen* both originated in the Old German word *draugmah*, which means "phantom," coming from the Indo-European *dreugh*, which means "to deceive." Furthermore, the association between the German *dreaming* (*traumarbeit*) and *trauma* is shown in the *Quartet*, particularly in regard to Durrell's statement on the healing power of writing. Writing within the realm of dreams allows Durrell to accomplish that which he deems impossible – to convert personal trauma into art. The language of dreams allows him to verbalise experiential elements that cannot be otherwise conceptualised. Early on in *Justine*, Darley writes of his wish to extract the living, sensory essence of his friends and weave them into the story of his memory. He wants them to awaken again to life so that he can create his story in their shape. Without clearly stating it, Durrell is describing what Freud referred to as *unheimliche*, where it is impossible to tell the living from the dead.[1] Thus, he hoped, he would be able to transform his pain into art. Even though success is far from guaranteed, he must try.[2] He continues to writes that he struggles to tell reality from dream when reflecting on his life in Alexandria, again echoing the sense of *unheimliche*. He points out that during the period in question, the dream experience overtook him and seemed to wipe out the actual experience of existence.

Durrell establishes the language of dreams as one of the central pillars of the story. The language of dreams serves both as a structure for the whole work and a content provider. For Durrell, the language of dreams is the medium wherein he processes his diverse, complex experiences, which form his mind as expressed in this work. The present chapter will draw upon the psychoanalytic concepts of the language of dreams in the interpretation of *The Alexandria Quartet* that inspired Durrell when writing and constructing the work.[3] Evidence of the importance that Durrell attributed to dreams and the dreaming process can be found early in his career, in a short essay he wrote in 1947, where he describes his and his colleagues' dreams during a joint tour of the Greek island of Kos. Durrell recounts how the entire tour was inspired by the dream experience and goes so far as to argue that the particular dream dreamt by one of his colleagues calls to mind the history of the place they have visited.[4]

In this chapter, two aspects of the dream language will be discussed. The first shows how the structure of the entire work can be interpreted as resting on the structure conception of the dream. The second is the use of particular dreams in the text to express particular themes: the vicissitudes of sexuality, truth, belonging and power. Two dreams are analysed: Mountolive's "sexual dream" and Nessim's "political dream". The use of dreams is anchored in the notion that it is a blurred line that runs between dream and reality in the reflective process of the individual when it comes to the question of *truth*. The images that surface in the dreams of the characters of the *Quartet* blend in with the images that emerge from their lives, to the extent that it is hard to tell dream from reality. The dream becomes no less, and perhaps even more, significant than reality in shaping the mind of the protagonists or narrative voices. As Darley claimed in *Clea*, the final volume, that it had become hard for him to leave the field of dreams where he felt he had resided in his mind in favour of the new experiences he had encountered upon his return to Alexandria. He found it impossible to keep the two apart – images from his dreams were interacting with real experiences, making it hard for him to tell them apart.[5]

The interpretation of dreams as an unconscious expression of the human mind is one of the pillars of psychoanalytic theory.[6] As previously noted, the dream itself (the text) is differentiated from the dream work (the text's interpretation). When listening to the story of the dream, we listen both to the conscious (manifest) and unconscious (latent) layers of the text. Freud's assumption was that the repressed contents of the unconscious will emerge in the dream through a complex system of filters (defence mechanisms), the very same ones through which the contents have been repressed in the first place. These defences include *displacement*, *condensation*, *sublimation* and *projection*, all of which can be detected through the text. An interpretation that bears in mind psychoanalytical insights allows reading\listening to the text in a manner that calls to mind the therapist who listens to the patient's unconscious contents.[7]

Freud was not the first thinker to invest the dream with meaning or to propose that we try to interpret it. Dreams have always formed a basis for writers to interpret conscious expressions, prophecies or mythical structures. Nor was Freud the first to argue that dreams reflected the repressed desires of the dreamer or that in order to interpret dreams one must follow the associations evoked in their wake.[8] Freud was unique in treating the prospect of interpreting dreams not as a mere symbolical display but rather as a crucial element in the therapeutic method he created to analyse the content of the mind of the individual. He established the theory of the dream on the three main frames of reference that had existed before him: the romantic approach, which saw the dream as a personal, ulterior manifestation of an inner desire, the rational approach, which viewed the manifest content of the dream as assorted expressions, and the somatic approach, which viewed the dream to be a mental manifestation of physical processes. Freud bound those three approaches together when he established the dream interpretation therapeutic method that relied on listening to the dream's story as told by the patient, and on the ensuing dream work. Psychoanalytic theory emphasises the possibility of interpreting words and actions in different, and even contradictory, ways, without compromising their vitality, veracity or validity. The same word, the same act, the very same figure, will attract different, seemingly contradictory interpretations, according to the manner and context of their presentation. Narrative truth holds true only relative to its speaker and context. In his short essay from 1910, "The Antithetical Meaning of Primal Words," Freud elaborates the idea he first presented ten years earlier in *The Interpretation of Dreams*. It concerns the characterisation ascribed by Freud to a dream that contains contradictory contents. This characterisation stems from the nature of language:

> The way in which dreams treat the category of contraries and contradictories is highly remarkable. It is simply disregarded. "No" seems not to exist so far as dreams are concerned. They show a particular preference for combining contraries into a unity or for representing them as one and the same thing. Dreams feel themselves at liberty, moreover, to represent any element by its wishful contrary; so that there is no way of deciding at a first glance whether any element that admits of a contrary is present in the dream-thoughts as a positive or as a negative.[9]

According to Freud, inspired by writings of philologist Carl Abel (1837–1906),[10] the dream can encompass contradictory meanings since language does the same. Freud quotes Abel, who demonstrates how in ancient languages like Egyptian (and Hebrew), the same word was used to describe one phenomenon and its antithesis.[11] With time, these *primal words* were transformed so that one phenomenon and its antithesis were assigned different words, even though their linguistic affinity remains evident. Freud describes how reading Abel's writings helped him overcome the hurdle of understanding the textual contradiction phenomenon in his patients' dreams, and indeed, in his own dreams. This revelation, as was also experienced in the *unheimliche* phenomena, amounted to a revolution for him, as it led him to the notion that the dream, and consequently the unconscious, were not driven and constructed based on rational, linear rules, but rather moulded after the dreamer's repressed wishes. The insight immediately ensues that the interpretation of dreams and texts alike cannot be objective; rather, they rest on the subjectivity of the dreamer and the interpreter.

Dream work, as described by the British psychoanalyst Christopher Bollas (born 1943), implies paying attention to the associations made by the patient following the story of the dream, which the psychoanalyst then links to previous insights that concern the patient.[12] Freud's ideas and their elaboration by analysts like Wilfred Bion (1897–1979), Donald Meltzer (1922–2004), James Grotstein

(1926–2015) and others, emphasised the centrality of the dream and dreaming process in the self's mental processes. The British psychoanalyst Thomas Ogden accordingly argues that the ability to dream and the ability to remember and relate the dream are the cornerstones upon which the subject's personality is founded.[13] Bion describes the dreaming process as part of a thinking mode that allows the individual's psyche to cope with emotional experiences and make sense of them, asserting that in order for the individual's everyday activity to have an impact, it must undergo some sort of dreaming process.[14] This notion, that the dreaming process itself, and the ensuing interpretive work, form part of the individual's reflective process has been recently explored by Israeli psychoanalyst Moshe Halevi Spero (born 1956) in his article on the dreams of biblical Joseph and Pharaoh. This study stresses that the dream process and its ensuing dream work allow the human psyche to create the mental framework where the subjects can bring together different parts of their personality and form cognitive and emotional continuums to connect between them.[15]

For the author of *The Alexandria Quartet*, the dream and dream work are a manifestation of his ambition to create awareness where imagination meets reality, in an encounter that involves conscious and unconscious layers, past memories and present experiences. For him, the return to the city, to the primordial experience through the act of writing, is the setting that creates the complete, undivided pattern of memory.[16] The narrator's overall memories and experiences, the memories buried in the unconscious layer of his psyche as well as experiences he is consciously aware of, establish his sense of self as moulded around a particular metaphoric pattern that has the city of Alexandria at its heart. All the contradictions that seem to have existed in his memory and dreams lose their sense of contrariness. The past and present have become a single entity that cannot be told apart, just as contradictions cannot be told apart in a dream.

The dream as a structure

The arrangement of the *Quartet*'s four volumes, their order of appearance, the different plots that follow from each volume to form the overall narrative fabric – all these are no coincidence. Durrell wrote each volume so as to reflect a particular aspect of the overall *mindscape* that he wanted to represent in the book as a whole.[17] Durrell presented the *Quartet* as if it was an individual whose depth and stratification of mind gradually unfolded for the reader. In a letter he wrote to Henry Miller while working on the tetralogy, Durrell described the structure he had designed as a stratified story with two layers of the same story that fit into each other, while another layer, the *orthodox* layer, encompasses them, interpenetrating the contents:

> The grand plan, if I can do it, is four books of which the first two fit into each another – different but the same book – Giordano Bruno! The next which I shall start after tea today is a big orthodox novella *interpenetrating* the two previous ones at many points![18]

The way that Durrell *interpenetrate* the different layers echo Freud's argument that dreams were formed from two intermingling elements: the first one is traces of the day that preceded the dream, the memories collected in the dreamer's consciousness. The second element is the emergence of unconscious contents, which attach themselves onto the memories of the previous day and by so doing transform, *interpenetrate*, their meaning. Thus, unconscious contents surface into awareness, combining elements from two realms, not unlike the way metaphors operate. New meaning can be understood and processed through dream work.[19] In the *Quartet*, as one progresses through reading the different layers of the story, the significance of the different characters and narrative voices changes in a similar way. New information, which arrives from what could be considered the unconscious realms of the novel, *interpenetrates* previous understanding and creates new meaning.

After first seeing Justine, Darley confesses in the first pages of the *Quartet*, he did not *dream* that she could be his lover, as she becomes later on.[20] After seeing her for the first time, he lies in bed, slowly entering the labyrinthine realm of dreams where he wanders, tortured by forbidden desire. Dreaming of Justine as his lover, and upon waking fearing the realisation of the dream, is a subtle clue as to the grave dangers Darley would indeed face once his wish comes true. The unconscious is filled with repressed wishes that are placed there, so to speak, in order to guard the dreamer from the unwarranted content that could put to risk his sense of stability and familiarity. The object of his desire remains barred from him, buried in deep regions of his consciousness. He dares not make such a move but succumbs to her initiative. When he does become her lover, his life changes. The fulfilment of the forbidden wish breaks down the boundaries. What was only unconscious has become conscious. The wish *interpenetrated* his awareness. But rather than bringing him a sense of satisfaction and achievement, it brings him danger. At the end, he has to flee Alexandria and finds refuge on a remote Greek island, licking his wounds.

Contemplating the events, Darley realises that the time he spent in Alexandria was time spent in a *dream*. Everybody behaved as if they were in the realm of dreams, where boundaries become blurred, where subjective reality becomes unstable and unreliable, where life is governed by the deepest, untamed impulses. Durrell stages the dream realm as a place where Darley cannot find peace. It is not confined to sleep, but floods his waking hours and creates a disruptive, disturbing existential experience. Even when awake, he questions the stability of his reality and struggles to decide whether or not he dreams. When faced with banal tasks, such as finding a taxi on the street, he describes his experience as the stuff of bad traumatic dreams. These are not just dreams, these are nightmares. He does not desire the dream, nor does he wish to understand it and be transformed by it. He wants to be awakened from it, so he can regain his sense of self. Alas, he is a prisoner of his own consciousness, dominated by contents he had wished he had never been exposed to. The *Quartet*'s first volume, *Justine*, is dominated by his associations as he tries to make sense of what had happened to him. He writes associatively, voicing his grievances and pain, seeking to be heard and be understood. In *Justine*, Darley is like the patient speaking with his therapist, hoping to find solace and sense, waiting for reassuring words that would allow him to regain his equilibrium.

Along his stream of associations, Darley's voice breaks into other narrative voices, like the voice of writer Jacob Arnauti, who was married to Justine years before Darley arrived in Alexandria. Darley receives a copy of the novel Arnauti wrote about his relationship with Justin (named Claudia in his book) and quotes from it at length. The bifurcation of the narrative voice reflects the structure of the novel and the paradox and contradiction Darley experiences when meeting Justine. Parts of him are split off and recede into deeper layers of his psyche. He moves into the realm of dreams. The new topography he has created is loose and resilient enough to encompass all those elements that Darley discovers in himself as a result of meeting Justine. He is unravelled by her, regressing into a primeval sense of himself where he is less sure of his boundaries. Following their encounter, and the internal experience thereby evoked, the new inner space that is created forces him to address deep existential issues. He is again thrown to face his sense of belonging, his loneliness, his *secret wound*. Through the words of Arnauti, Darley emerges from the realm of the dream. Through the knowledge of what Justine *really* wanted from him, he is able, and forced to integrate the new experience into his world. It is through the act of writing that he hopes he would be able to put all the pieces back together. The book that he imagines will not be a regular book. The plot, or content, would not be significant. What would matter would be the form itself. The writing of the book would be like re-creating his home, which would then contain his newly acquired ability to dream.

The second volume, *Balthazar*, introduces another layer into the realm of dream. During work on this volume, Durrell often referred to it as *Justine 2*, while its final name was given to it relatively late into the work. This book reveals further facts concerning the first book's events, recasting them in a new light. In fact, this book mostly comprises an interpretation of the first book by Dr. Balthazar, who pays a visit to Darley on his Greek island exile and offers his comments on the first book, *the interlinear*. This volume plants the seed of doubt regarding the reliability of *truth* as presented in the first volume. The narrator is no longer certain of the veracity of his own version of events. The reality exposed by Balthazar seems to undermine Darley's worldview and compromises his ability to trust the validity and authenticity of his own experiences and existence. This volume poses a challenge to Darley's view of the world as a stable place where events are what they seem. It suddenly dawns on the narrator that he is not the master of his own destiny as he fancied himself to be. He understands that his actions are not really the product of his free will and the romantic setting he has made for himself, but are rather manipulated and controlled by other, greater powers, of which he is unaware.

The poignant remarks made by Balthazar form the interpretation (dream work) of the volume written by Darley in his exile (the dream). Not unlike an interpretation made by a psychoanalyst, the interpretation made by Balthazar stirs a mixed response in Darley. On the one hand, he is relieved, feeling that new horizons have opened up for him as far as understanding his actions and emotional experiences.

On the other hand, he has a sense of pain and loss as he is no longer able to maintain his romantic worldview, which facilitated his sensory, tempestuous infatuation with Justine. His disillusionment following Balthazar's interpretation is the first in a series of disillusionments that lie ahead for him.

If the first two volumes can be likened to the dream and dream work, the third volume, *Mountolive*, marks the moment of awakening from the dream. The volume's opening page cites Marquis de Sade's (1740–1814) *Justine, or The Misfortunes of Virtue*. In this excerpt, Durrell points to that moment of awakening or disillusion from a dream, when the dreamer dreams no more and becomes aware of the contents he has just dreamt in his sleep:

> The dream dissipated, were one to recover one's common sense mood, the thing would be of but mediocre import – 'tis the story of mental wrongdoing. Everyone knows very well and it offends no one. But alas! One sometimes carries the thing a little further. What, one dares wonder, what would not be the idea's realization if its mere abstract shape thus exalted has just so profoundly moved one? The accursed reverie is vivified and its existence is a crime.[21]

Durrell quotes de Sade, who writes that the dream dissipated, leaving behind a moral question: what must the dreamer do when the content of his dream betrays to him his forbidden wishes and the prospect of realising them? The question's phrasing indicates that de Sade found it futile to dream arousing contents per se. Once the dreamer has experienced these contents in the dream, his path is paved to realise them in practice, even if this entails a crime. He is ruined. It is therefore not surprising that in the third volume of the *Quartet*, the narrative voice of Darley disappears. *Mountolive* is cast as re-telling the story that recurred in the first two volumes, but this time objectively, in a manner that lays bare its subjective bias. The same existential realities that were presented in the first two volumes as words of truth will be recast in the third volume in an *objective* light. The story might remain the same, but will no longer be submerged in the realm of dreaming: the characters of the *Quartet* are portrayed as they *really* are; corrupt, weak, human. The author in this volume is no longer the dreamy, innocent narrative voice of the two previous volumes: Darley makes way for an anonymous narrative voice, who is not identified by name and does not play a part in the plot. He remains outside of it, telling the story *as is*. *Mountolive* embodies the objective layer of the story (*orthodox*, as Durrell refers to it). But this objective side is in fact the convergence of the different layers of the mind of the author. No longer trapped in the romantic perception that marks the first volume or in the disillusionment of the second one, the narrator now inhabits a new, seemingly mature position, which pulls together the different split-off layers of his mind. This moment marks the return of the narrator to reckon with the real circumstances of his life. It is the moment of *insight*, when he sees and understands consciously what had been so far only insinuated. As in therapy, it is the moment when the patient realises and understands something significant in his life. It is an insight that *makes sense* of all that had been till then mysterious and troubling. It is perhaps a moment of painful realisation, but it bears great clarity and even hope for a future which may reveal the Sisyphean cycles that life had been so far.

The fourth volume, *Clea*, sees Darley resuming the position of the main narrator. Described by Durrell as the sequel of *Justine*, it is indeed the linear continuation of the plot laid out in the first volume. It is the volume of return to the place that Durrell describes in the first volume. *Clea* sees Darley return to Alexandria after an absence of a few years to meet the still living characters that were present in the first volume. It is Durrell's homecoming tale, his return to his imaginary homeland. It is here that Darley gathers all the insights he has gained over the years of exile. He is still pondering the complexity and richness of inner sights that staying in the realm of dreams has given him.[22] His return to Alexandria is not an ordinary return. Despite his changed awareness, he is still driven by a force unknown to him. He has come to repair an inner wound. He is returning to the scene of the primal experience, the place where he experienced his rite of passage. He must return to Alexandria because he has never actually managed to leave it. His experience of belonging to the city, characterised at once as an empowering dream and a shattering traumatic experience, leaves him as a pawn in the hands of greater powers. He must return to the city, because he is a part of it. The actual return to the city is a metaphoric return to his own self, that is, acknowledgement of the split parts of his mind. The return to the city, following his disillusionment with the dream, is the attempt to reclaim and gather together his shattered mind.

Durrell acknowledged the power of the dream to access the deeper layers of the mind. He was also aware how elusive such a descent can be, how resistant is the mind to let go of its old repetitive defensive mechanism. Through the voice of Balthazar, he declares that the contents of the mind which are protected by a psychic defence mechanism will not be revealed easily. The *truth* will have to be forced out, through dreams.[23] Is there such a truth, he wonders? In writing *The Alexandria Quartet*, Durrell sought to show how different parts of the mind experienced reality and truth in different fashions. In order to show that no given version of the story was necessarily the exclusively true version, Durrell developed the structure of the *Quartet* to gradually expose the reader to the complexities of the story, using different perspectives. Durrell does not venture to generate a flattening, sweeping gaze on the story, but rather leaves the reader with different options of understanding the plot and characters. By so doing, he keeps the work in the realm of dreams, where any unequivocal, consistent and solid interpretation is rejected; it is always subjected to different, varying interpretations. As succinctly put by Freud: "Dreams, like all other psychopathological structures, regularly have more than one meaning."[24] The instability of *truth* is a result of the precarious relation between the manifest and latent contents of the mind. It changes according to the course of reading the text, or listening to the patient as exemplified by the Freudian term *nachträglich,* referred to in the first chapter, denoting a current understanding which changes the perception of the past. Thus, that which appeared at first to be manifest and *true*, later transpires to be more complicated due to the latent content which became manifest in *Balthazar*. The process continues into the third volume, *Mountolive*, where reading renders the content of the first two volumes manifest, while the latent content is contained in *Mountolive*. This confusing experience generates disorientation, which makes it hard for the reader to decide where the manifest or latent content of the *Quartet* is. The fourth volume attempts to bring the reader to a more certain, rational and linear position regarding what is true and what is not. Following the narrative upheavals of the three previous volumes, this volume is the conclusion of the *Quartet*. Though not conclusive, the end allows the story to achieve some closure, when the reader is able to witness what could appear to be the end of the story. Still, the very last words of the *Quartet* are followed with a question mark, suggesting that even the end is not quite what it appears to be. As I suggested in the previous chapter, the reader is left to decide for himself whether the story will continue or not.

Mountolive's dream

In the following pages I will study two of the dreams that appear in the *Quartet* to show how Durrell used *dream* and *dream work* to illustrate the multi-layered nature of the work. The first dream I will explore appears in *Mountolive*. It is the dream of Mountolive whose perspective delivers the "realistic" version of events in Alexandria. The dream described by the anonymous narrator features a childhood scene from Mountolive's life. In the dream, Mountolive is with his mother as she reads aloud to him from Jonathan Swift's (1667–1745) *Gulliver's Travels*. Mountolive dreams the dream while he is semi forced to stay at a brothel in Alexandria. The dream, which he literally falls into, happens when he finds himself surrounded by a group of children held there for the gratification of adults. I suggest that the dream is introduced at that stage to prevent Mountolive from having sexual contact with the children. At the height of his confusion and intoxication (he had drunk several glasses of *arak* by then), he enters a heightened state of consciousness and dreams of the time his mother read to him from the book which was illustrated with large colour-plates depicting Gulliver in the hands of the little people of Lilliput.[25] Mountolive found himself in the presence of child prostitutes after he wandered off from the Alexandrian street to a shop where he began talking to the proprietor and then led him into the inner recesses of the establishment. Inside he is given a drink of *arak* by a "shiek," misinterpreting, deliberately or not, the wish and desire of the white British foreigner who wandered into his establishment. Durrell portrays Mountolive as someone who has found himself in the brothel by accident, but once inside, surrounded by a group of naked children, his faculties are clouded. It is his loss of consciousness and the ensuing dream that spares him from sexual contact with the children.

Durrell constructed the dream relying on the formula Freud suggested: a mixture between the remains of the day, a current strong evocative experience, driven by powerful, repressed (sexual) drive. Durrell employed some ingenuity in suggesting that the dream experience did not have to happen while the dreamer was actually asleep. It was enough that he felt threatened by his present surroundings, and current state of mind, to slip into that altered-consciousness state. In my view, Durrell thus suggested that dreaming indeed saved Mountolive from succumbing to deeply buried sexual fantasies. The dream serves as *a transitional experience* that protects him. But the dream is not without its impressions of those palpable experiences that Mountolive tries to escape. He seems to revert to a sheltered primeval experience where his mother reads Swift's book to him, but even within the dream he finds no peace, as this particular dream recreates parts of the scene he tried to escape and he finds himself surrounded by little people who bind him to the ground. In that, Durrell suggests that the dream was only partially successful in guarding Mountolive from the repressed contents of his unconscious.

Mountolive finds that his being had been altered following that event and the dream, and he can no longer regain his peace of mind. He has to leave. It is only through this departure that he imagines he could break free from the shackles of the City, which exerts powers that he finds himself helpless against, particularly when facing deep impulses of which he has not been aware. It is the City that stirred up the forbidden sexual desires that materialise simultaneously in his life and dream. No longer can he tell what came first – the dream scene with his mother reading him the tale of Gulliver in the land of Lilliput, or that horror scene in the brothel, where he found himself almost overpowered by a host of children. He feels he can no longer trust himself. Having had his consciousness altered following the dream, he feels he must change, and search for another posting.

Durrell portrayed the dream experience as having had a dual impact: on the one hand it did protect Mountolive from his repressed, forbidden sexual impulses, but, since that protection was not complete, he can never trust reality in the same way he had. In that sense, Durrell portrays Mountolive as someone who had experienced a trauma and is now dealing with its mental and emotional consequences. The dream was the safe space where Mountolive could encounter the forbidden parts of his mind in a manner that guards him against committing perverse sexual acts. However, the very act of dreaming and remembering altered his consciousness. The encounter with the unfamiliar and forbidden, the *unheimliche*, conjures up the affinity with the primeval place that has protected him from such experiences, the presence of his mother. But as his defences are already breached, he can no longer revert to the same innocent place. It is lost for him. Nevertheless, his wish to return to a primeval – though different – experience is not lost. Durrell portrayed the dream as a reflective process that alters the mind of the dreamer and drives him towards a real change in life, based on the newly gained understanding. It is suggested by my reading of the text that Mountolive can no longer continue as if nothing had happened, having realised he harbours those perverse sexual urges. Even if he has not acted upon them and succeeds in sublimating his urges – as proven by the dream, he is no longer the same person. The dream has saved Mountolive from becoming a sexual offender, but could not save him from himself, from coming face to face with his forbidden urges: Mountolive emerges from the dream a different person. The world is still familiar but it is actually this familiarity that he finds disturbing. It is *unheimliche*. It holds a secret that for the time being haunts him.[26]

Nessim's dream

Durrell uses another dream earlier in the *Quartet* to represent yet another theme. This is a dream dreamt by Nessim Hosnani, Justine's husband. Nessim plays a twofold part in *Justine*, both a protagonist and a narrative voice. Mostly, he is portrayed as a tormented figure – Justine's betrayed husband – but towards the middle of the volume, he becomes a narrative voice. This ploy of changing the identity of the narrative voice seems to take place randomly, almost unwittingly. It is not the first time that the identity of the narrative voice changes in the course of the plot. As discussed in the second chapter, Durrell created a choir of narrative voices deliberately. It was his conviction that the narrative voice cannot be a single, continuous voice, but rather a multiplicity of voices, to reflect the nature and structure of the human mind. Unlike previous occasions, this time when the shift between the different narrative voices takes place, it happens unannounced, with no explanation, Nessim's voice appears out of the blue, seemingly barging into the story. Nessim assumes, and then abandons, the narrative voice abruptly, with neither explanation nor a justified plot development to account for his move. The entire scene is like an episode in a dream that makes no logical or linear association with whatever comes before or after. An attempt to follow the course of the dream will leave the readers perplexed, sending them into a reflective, speculative process, as is the experience of reading this part of the story, leaving a sense of disorientation and bewilderment. The author plants this episode as an association. At this point in the story, the episode remains obscure and troubling. It is only as the plot develops that it acquires a broader context, which casts a new, much more significant light on it.

The first reference to the dream appears early on in *Justine* when it is mentioned that Nessim is again dreaming of his childhood. The dreams are described as disturbing as they preoccupy him and disrupt his ordinary goings-on. No mention at this point is made in reference to the actual content of the dream. Nessim's dream, which takes him back to a childhood scene, speaks to an early life experience left unaddressed. The disturbing memory seeks resolution. It is not just any dream that the narrator recounts. The experience endured by Nessim is a disturbing one. He is assailed by the dream, with an unconscious content that seeks outlet in his consciousness. It is Nessim's mission to express this urge, in order to maintain his mental health. The disturbing dream intimidates him, tearing into his life.

This childhood dream soon make way for other dreams which do not refer to his childhood. They appear not as a device to resolve a painful personal conflict. They are replaced by *historical* dreams, thus stating that Nessim's cultural belonging far exceeds his personal or even familial ties. In this instance, Durrell attributes a different weight to the significance of the dream. It is no longer a dream representing the inner world of the individual. The interpretation of the dream pertains to the collective memory of the community the dreamer is a part of. This characterisation of the dream diverges from Freud's interpretation of dreams and is inspired by the ideas of the Swiss psychologist Carl Jung.[27] According to Jung, dreams can represent a collective psyche of a group of people who share some communal heritage, as well as the individual psyche of particular individuals.

The idea that the dream contains historical truth which is beyond any individual significance is a key motive in plot of *The Alexandria Quartet*. As the very same dream can be interpreted either way, the path that Durrell points to at this stage, suggests that the individual himself carries no overwhelming significance, but rather serves as an insignificant, expendable detail. Darley's romantic escapades, therefore, are not as substantial as may have transpired from the chapters that precede the dream. Darley's dalliances, his infatuation with Justine, his relationships with his colleagues at the British Embassy and scores of other details, all these decrease in specific gravity relative to the collective historical truth that Nessim hints at when describing the dream process.[28] Nessim calls upon the reader to delve deeper into the text and pay attention to an historical layer that was hidden earlier by the sentimentality that the earlier childhood dreams evoked. This focus again uses Freudian ideas regarding manifest and latent layers in the dream. What had first appeared to be a story of a private individual (manifest) appears to be a story of a collective community (latent). As specified in chapter four, where I discuss the role of the city of Alexandria as *a poetic space*, Nessim cites the city as an arena where this oscillation between the private and collective realms of the dream is enacted. Durrell places these two aspects in a dichotomy as part of the existential journey of the protagonist. He addresses the readers, asking that they look at the historical aspects of his existence rather than focus on all those romantic, individual particulars that filled the book until then. He asks the readers to rise above their identification with the main protagonist, Darley, and pay attention to another, deeper-lying layer, which he seeks to assert in the story, by describing Nessim's dreaming process.

The meaning of the historical dreams slowly transpires. Nessim's historical dream is a dream of return. To achieve that he strikes a political pact with Justine. But it is not a return to one's homeland. This is not the exiled individual's return to the primeval space of his early life. The return that Nessim dreams, with an intensity that paralyses him through the greater part of the *Quartet*'s third volume, is a collective return of a nation to its *unheimliche* homeland. Yet even the pact with Justine does not necessarily lead to the longed-for liberation and return. In line with the organising principle of the entire work, each of the protagonists, including Nessim, realises repeatedly that his volition is not strong enough to turn the wheels of history. His actions are forever countered with stronger forces that put him in his place.

What is the greater historical move that Nessim hints at, which pits the fate of the individual against greater powers? The *Quartet*'s first two volumes see the characters preoccupied with interpersonal tangles, and in so doing Durrell has moulded them as modern protagonists preoccupied with issues of existence, self-fulfilment and love. But in the last two volumes of the work, he incorporates another element, which turns the picture on its head. Nessim's dream concerns his wish to reinstate the Coptic minority to power in Egypt and subvert the Muslims' overtaking of his country. This is no imaginary return to a lost mother but a political return to power within the same country that has been taken from the Coptic minority with the pact struck between the British colonisers and the Muslim majority. As discussed in chapter five, it is doubtful whether Lawrence Durrell really intended to describe the power relations between the Copts, the Muslims and British. Michael Haag suggests that the events Durrell described in the *Quartet* were meant to disguise the fact that what was really being described was the efforts of the Jewish underground in British Mandated Palestine to purchase arms in Egypt with the help of the Jewish community in Alexandria, particularly the Menasce family (to whom his third wife was related).[29] But in order to protect the family members, who at the time of the *Quartet*'s writing in the 1950s, were still residing in the city, from the regime's wrath, Durrell changed the identity of the conspirators. However, this does not alter the governing principle: it is the greater power, the City of Alexandria that controls the lives of the people who reside in it, regardless of their individual actions. The subjective intentions of the characters are but a drop in the ocean of latent powers seething in the *oceanic* layers of the City.

The political undercurrent revealed to the reader in *Mountolive* draws on actual events from that period. This rallying of the Coptic minority in Egypt that Durrell described tried to prevent the Muslim majority from stepping into the governing vacuum left by the end of the British rule in Egypt. The country's Coptic minority, fearing the Muslims' rise with the British retreat, tried to establish ties with the Jewish underground organisations in Palestine, with the purpose of selling them arms.[30] These arms were meant to reinforce the Jewish struggle for independence, waged against the British forces. The Copts were hoping that the victory of the Zionist movement and the founding of the State of Israel would constitute an incentive for their struggle against the Muslim overtaking of the local government in Egypt, and that a strategic alliance would be formed between the Jewish state and Egypt's Coptic community against the region's Muslim forces. This is clearly stated by Nessim in *Justine* when he says to Justine, as part of their pact-making, that there was only one nation that can change the course of events in the Middle East. He declares that only the Jews, as the eternal dispossessed foreigners, will be able to help the Copts gain their independence in Egypt.[31]

Durrell spans the plot of the *Quartet* on the basis of the secret pact between Nessim and Justine. At the heart of it stands Nessim, the head of the powerful Coptic Hosnani family. He marries Jewish Justine, who assists him in executing his plan. Justine's liaisons with Darley and others are designed to make sure the scheme is kept a secret and undisturbed by the British presence in Egypt. All her dalliances are towards this single end. *Modern love*, the purported theme of the *Quartet*, transpires as defence and disguise for the real scheme. Once this scheme is exposed and thwarted, Darley, and the readers, are faced with a picture that is altogether different from the one offered at the beginning. *Modern love* emerges as political ruse. The *modern love* that the book delves into transpires as a screen drawn over a political story. *Modern love* is the manifest content while the political activity is the latent content of the *Quartet*. The passion shown by Justine and Nessim is not about consummating their love but rather about realising their political ambitions of forging affinity between two minorities – the Copts in Egypt and the Jews in Palestine. The key question, as it turns out, is not just the existential voyage of the protagonist, nor the interpersonal relations between the protagonists, but also the issue of their belonging to a greater collective experience.

The issue of belonging is vital to the entire work and acts in it as an organising principle. As Israeli historian Ella Belfer writes:

> The notion of collective identity is a key one in the postmodern world where globalization and tribalization interplay as social trends in modern day multicultural society. The more fluid and unstable the values of the individual become, so the collective impact of the universal values rises. As the big singular answers to life's existential dilemma dissolve, so the quest for a firmer sense of belonging becomes more urgent.[32]

Durrell, exile at heart and with no clear geographical and cultural sense of belonging, understood that the existential issues that the individual deals with are incomplete without bringing in his sense of belonging to a community. A man is not an island, even if he escapes to one every now and then. Being biologically and culturally part of any one community is a simple fact and does not settle the issue of belonging.

Durrell was sensitive both to the aspirations of the Copts in Egypt and the Jews in Palestine, partly because he had spent the years that preceded his work on the *Quartet* working for the British administration, and was aware of the different political movements in the countries where he had served. The independence aspirations of the Jews, on the one hand, and the Copts, on the other, reflected his childhood in India, in its struggle for independence from British colonial rule. As I have emphasised throughout the book, the best term I find to describe Durrell's relation to a homeland, actual or imaginary, is embodied in the term *unheimliche*. He felt both at home and a stranger in any of the places he had resided in. His birthplace in India remained an Eden that he was expelled from by his paternal command at the age of eleven. England, which could be considered his ancestral homeland, evoked in him strong ambivalent feelings. Greece offered him a temporary home where he found his literary voice. He finally settled in France, where he could lead his chosen life style while never completely abandoning his passion for Greece and often returning to it. His home was in his writing. The complex question of belonging could not be resolved by settling in one part of the world or another. The conflicts at play between his longing for the primordial experience of life as child in India and his ambivalence towards the Anglo-Saxon culture, the object of his ancestors' aspirations, were relentless, and acted as a major driving force in his work.

The manifest aspects of this conflict were seen in his travelling around the world. The latent aspects were shown in his relationships with women which became the place to which he aspired to belong and sought to find a home. Through Nessim's dream, he confesses that it was the woman who is the key figure in the power relations he described. Nessim attributes to her political aspirations which are the underlying driving force behind all her actions, including her behaviour in love.[33] Nessim turns our attention to the complex meaning of *modern love*, which was declared as the key theme of the entire work. But even this term, *modern love*, stands as a screen for the real concern, which is the issue of feminine sexuality and its role in charting the actual power relations in reality. That is *the truth* about the woman.[34] Her real power lies in her ability to operate under the veil bestowed on her by romantic culture. Her romantic figure is the perfect guise. The sensuality that serves her as a façade to the world is in fact a mask behind which the deep powers that drive the wheels of culture, wars and history huddle together. At the end of the day, it is these greater powers which will not let the individual follow his own heart. Whenever he thinks he may break free of the shackles that rob him of his creativity, he realises that the freedom he has gained is in fact a new setting that closes on him again.[35] Try as he might, Durrell cannot envisage at this stage a world where the individual is really free of this sense of belonging to an oppressive homeland. He will continue to search and maybe even recreate his sense of belonging. It is a quest for what had been lost. It is the search that is a major driving force in his motivation as a writer. The missing homeland experience guides Durrell in his quest for a place he can call home.

Dreams and the aspiration for truth

The narrative turn in the story of the *Quartet* brought by Nessim's dream represents a claim for truth which is contradictory to the original claim of writing a work where there is no single particular truth. What is revealed through the dream implies that there *is* a single truth underlying the actions of the protagonists in the book, even if it remains buried. Truth is no longer multifaceted nor relative, as argued in the prefatory notes; truth lies in a place deep down that must be striven towards. Truth, therefore, is not a reflection of the perspective of the individual, but exists as a very particular essence that can be uncovered with the appropriate method. In his 1937 essay, *Constructions in Analysis*, Freud illustrated his concept of truth by drawing an analogy between the efforts the analyst makes to the work of the archaeologist. Both assume that there is always another layer of testimonial experience buried underneath what is visible. The truth as such can never be completely discovered but only added to. "His work of construction, or, if it is preferred, of reconstruction, resembles to a great extent an archaeologist's excavation of some dwelling-place that has been destroyed and buried or of some ancient edifice."[36] In introducing Nessim's dream, Durrell declares that truth is a vestige of an ancient structure that can be excavated and uncovered in due course. It is no coincidence that Durrell employs a metaphor similar to Freud's. For him, the uncovering of the truth is tantamount to finding one's homeland. The search for the truth, and for the homeland, are inner voyages into his mind. All he has to do is venture into the depths of his consciousness so as to find the truth there.

To conclude, I suggest adopting the distinction made by the philosopher W.H. Walsh (1913–1986), who drew a distinction between the issue of *historical truth* –

the objective facts of subjective experience as independently existing prior to their verbal utterance by the subject – and the issue of *narrative truth*, defined as the account of facts as the part of the reflective process of the individual.[37] The psychoanalyst Donald Spence added that, since the most fundamental subjective experiences are formed in a preverbal stage of human development, any attempt to express those experiences in words as a single *truth* will be met with great difficulty.[38] Spence went further and stated that the *true* experiences that formed the identity of the individual, including their ability to recall them, could not be verbally expressed at all. According to him, it is those very experiences that will remain outside the realm of language. They may form *the truth* that we cannot discover, but can aspire towards.

Darley strives to uncover *truth*. His aspiration for truth sets him on a personal quest that can never end, and keeps sending him back to the starting point, as he writes in the opening pages of *Balthazar*, recalling his friend's warning that truth is often that which contradicts itself.[39] In *The Alexandria Quartet* Durrell planted *historical truth* within the realm of the dream language, or the *narrative truth*, of the entire work. The dream served Durrell as the turning key through which he tries to reconcile the inherently contradictory aspects of truth. It is only in the language of dreams that such a paradox can exist. The paradoxical and contradictory *truth* of the *Quartet*, claiming that the destiny of the individual is in the hands of greater powers, is represented both in the structure of the book and in the dreams described. Truth is to be found in the imagination of the author. It is found as an inner experience that guides him ahead in the Sisyphean path. Trying to act upon what seems to be true, leads the protagonist again and again to the painful recognition that he is not the master of his own destiny. Truth appears often as complex and paradoxical, often having no validation in reality. But the aspiration to keep adhering to the truth, alongside the willingness to acknowledge mistakes, is man's greatest drive in the creative course of his life. Man's ability to imagine relies on his ability in turn to keep acting upon what he deems true, even if he realises his errors time and again. Furthermore, it is the ability of the writer to rewrite himself again and again in light of what he keeps discovering through the act of writing, that makes writing the significant activity that it is.

Durrell makes no effort to reconcile the contradiction that appears between his statement in the prefatory notes about the absence of any exclusive truth and the way in which he constructs the entire plot as a path to discover a singular truth. The contradiction stands as evidence of his own state of mind and sense of being in the world. The lack of order or even sense, and even the contempt for order embodied by this contradiction, is another authentic manifestation of his irreparably split inner world. The unsettling *unheimliche* experience that may be generated within the reader does not worry the author in the body of the work, but he tries to resolve it with the workpoints that conclude each of the volumes (except *Mountolive*): the readers are free to continue the book as they will. The author holds no monopoly over the course that this work may take.

Notes

1 Freud, Sigmund, 1919, "The Uncanny", in J. Strachey, ed., *The Standard Edition of the Complete Psychological Works of Sigmund Freud*, trans. J. Strachey, Vol. XVII, London: Hogarth Press, pp. 217–252.
2 Durrell, Lawrence, 1957a, *Justine*, London: Faber & Faber, p. 17.
3 A clear distinction can be made between the dream which is the experience one has during the night, including its recall, however partial and fragmentary, and the dream work which is the interpretive associative analysis performed with the text of the dream, either in psychoanalytic work or through artistic endeavour, or simply in recalling its contents.
4 Durrell, Lawrence, 1947b, "Can Dreams Live on When Dreamers Die?" *The Listener*, September 25.
5 Durrell, Lawrence, 1960, *Clea*, London: Faber & Faber, pp. 12–13.
6 Freud, Sigmund, 1900, "The Interpretation of Dreams", in J. Strachey, ed., *The Standard Edition of the Complete Psychological Works of Sigmund Freud*, trans. J. Strachey, Vols. IV & V, London: Hogarth Press.
7 For further reading concerning the type of listening to the unconscious, I would refer the reader to Christopher Bollas (born 1943), himself a psychoanalyst from a literary background in his book published in 2007, Bollas, Christopher, *The Freudian Moment*, London: Karnac Books, pp. 33–65.
8 Aristo, for one, wrote that the most adept interpreter of dreams was the man who connected the parts of the dream and its ensuing verbal contents in the subject.
9 Freud, Sigmund, 1900, "The Interpretation of Dreams", in J. Strachey, ed., *The Standard Edition of the Complete Psychological Works of Sigmund Freud,* trans. J. Strachey, Vol. IV, London: Hogarth Press, p. 318.
10 Carl Abel was a German philologist who lived in Berlin and Oxford. He gained his renown mostly after publishing a voluminous dictionary in 1884, which explored the relations between the ancient Semitic language, particularly Egyptian, and the Anglo-Indian languages.
11 Spero, Moshe Halevi, 2018, "The Unique Contribution of Hebrew to the Conceptualization of the Psychodynamic Psychotherapy", in Rony Alfandary, ed., *Seeking Psychic Space: Fundamentals of Psychodynamic Social Work, (Hebrew)*, Jerusalem: Carmel Publishers, pp. 291–322.
12 Bollas, Christopher, 1991, *Forces of Destiny*, London: Association University Books, pp. 93–117.
13 Ogden, Thomas, 2003, "On Not Being Able to Dream", in *This Art of Psychoanalysis: Dreaming Undreamt Dreams and Interrupted Cries*, London & New York: Routledge, pp. 45–60.
14 Bion, Wilfred R., 1963, *Elements of Psycho-Analysis*, London: Maresfield and Karnac Books, pp. 65–90.
15 Spero, Moshe Halevi, 2010, "The Transformations in the 'Mental Apparatus of Dreaming' as Depicted in the Biblical Story of Joseph (Genesis 40–43)", in L. Aron and Libby Henik, eds., *Contemporary Psychoanalysis and Judaism*, New York: Academic Studies Press, p. 186.
16 Durrell, Lawrence, 1960, *Clea*, London: Faber & Faber, p. 91.
17 Pine, Richard, 2005, *Lawrence Durrell: The Mindscape*, Corfu: Durrell School of Corfu.
18 Durrell reference to Giordano Bruno, though a digression, is an example of his associative writing, inspired by his abundant reading. The casual tone fails to mask the grandiosity of his intention implied by the reference. The sixteenth-century Italian Catholic priest, Giordano Bruno (1548–1600), was executed by the Inquisition in Rome after refusing to renounce his convictions. Bruno made several claims that enraged the Catholic Church. He is considered by many to be the first man to sacrifice himself for science, preceding his contemporary Galileo, who also inherited his seat in Padova. Bruno's main claim that captivated Durrell's imagination was that the universe was neither uniform

nor unique but rather made of multiple parallel universes where the same event recurred in different versions, which were at once complementary and contradictory. MacNiven, Ian S., ed. 1988, *The Durrell-Miller Letters, 1935–1980*, London: Faber & Faber, p. 287.

19 Hodes, Matthew, 1989, "Dreams Reconsidered", *Anthropology Today*, 5:6–8; Hoffman, Frederick, 1945, *Freudianism and the Literary, Mind*, Baton Rouge: Louisiana State University Press.

20 Durrell, Lawrence, 1957a, *Justine*, London: Faber & Faber, p. 18.

21 De Sade, Marquis, 1965, *Justine or the Misfortunes of Virtue*, New York: Grove Press, p. 10.

22 Durrell, Lawrence, 1960, *Clea*, London: Faber & Faber, p. 55.

23 Durrell, Lawrence, 1958a, *Balthazar*, London: Faber & Faber, p. 148.

24 Freud, Sigmund, 1900, "The Interpretation of Dreams", in J. Strachey, ed., *The Standard Edition of the Complete Psychological Works of Sigmund Freud*, trans. J. Strachey, Vol. V, London: Hogarth Press, p. 149.

25 Durrell, Lawrence, 1958b, *Mountolive*, London: Faber & Faber, p. 293.

26 Ibid., p. 298.

27 Jung was one of Freud's closest colleagues at first but founded his own movement after he parted ways from Freud. The main disagreement between the two was Freud's insistence on the centrality of the sexual drive in determining the developmental course of the individual. For further reading: Jung, Carl, 1983, *Selected Writing*, ed. Anthony Storr, London: Fontana Press.

28 Durrell, Lawrence, 1957a, *Justine*, London: Faber & Faber, p. 140.

29 Manesce is the spelling that MacNiven uses in his biography. A more contemporary spelling of the Hebrew name is Menashe or Manasseh.

30 Egypt remained a British Protectorate until 1953.

31 Durrell, Lawrence, 1958b, *Mountolive*, London: Faber & Faber, p. 200.

32 Belfer, Ella, 2004, *A Split Identity: The Conflict between the Sacred and the Secular in the Jewish World (Hebrew)*, Ramat-Gan: Bar-Ilan University Press, p. 7.

33 Durrell, Lawrence, 1958b, *Mountolive*, London: Faber & Faber, p. 202.

34 The view expressed here towards "the woman" and towards women in general will be explored critically in later chapters.

35 Durrell, Lawrence, 1958b, *Mountolive*, London: Faber & Faber, p. 216.

36 Freud, Sigmund, 1937, "Constructions in Analysis", in J. Strachey, ed., *The Standard Edition of the Complete Psychological Works of Sigmund Freud*, trans. J. Strachey, Vol. XXIII, London: Hogarth Press, p. 259.

37 Walsh, W. H., 1958, "Plain and Significant Narrative," *History Journal of Philosophy*, 55:479–484.

38 Spence, Donald, 1982, *Narrative Truth and Historical Truth*, New York: W. W. Norton & Company Inc.

39 Durrell, Lawrence, 1958a, *Balthazar*, London: Faber & Faber, p. 23.

4

THE TOPOGRAPHIC RETURN TO THE MOTHER-CITY

Writing about the city of Alexandria, about arriving, staying, leaving and returning to the city, is at the heart of Durrell's experience of belonging, fictionally or concretely, to a particular physical place which can be called home. In the spirit of Steiner's words about the tragic fate of the individual to forever seek his fate in his journey towards his death, I will describe the process of writing as his way of dealing with the sense of death and loss of the mythical, primeval experience of belonging to a homeland, however fraught with difficulty and ambiguity that home was.[1] As Darley writes when trying to recapture his experience in the city, the mere mention of its name was like a reminder of the death he encountered in its presence.[2] Writing about Alexandria served Durrell as a mourning ritual, trying to return to a lost place and at the same time accept its demise. At the heart of Durrell's sense of belonging is his exilic experience. Writing about Alexandria created the internal arena where he could explore the ways in which the connection between the individual and his surroundings is both an integrative and deconstructive process. The sense of belonging that Durrell investigates is one where he feels predominantly alienated, helpless and even mortally threatened. Observing these impressions is akin to wandering through the city of the mind, as Haviva Pedaya wrote when describing the experience of searching for one's place:

> The deeper we explore the roots of exile-as-a-ritual we will see that it has something to do with walking in the city . . . the tension between walking towards a place in the city and aimless, restless wandering from one place to another.[3]

In the following pages, I shall follow Durrell's virtual and real footsteps through Alexandria, both as the actual city and as the fictional and liminal city it had become through his writing.

Durrell's actual experience in Alexandria, where he fled with the onset of the Second World War, served as his inspiration to establish the city's cosmopolitan urban space as a transitional and liminal experience in his life. The essence of this transitional experience lies in sexual experiences that the author portrays as a manifestation of the existential sickness that afflicts an individual who has strayed away from his connection with his homeland. Sexuality, which at first establishes one's hope of making sense of life through his romantic relations with women, emerges as the root of his sickness. The initially liberating, empowering sensual experience ends up subjecting him to debasing relations with women, whose sexuality is perceived as a harmful element that must be guarded against.

The city is also a transcendental being that subjugates one's consciousness. During his time in Alexandria, Durrell endured a personal crisis that pertained both to his marriage and his sense of belonging. Processing his personal experiences of the period through his writing provided him with a stage upon which he can express his ideas regarding one's identity in the face of his surroundings. The main thrust is that man was not master of his destiny, but was forced to persevere in his struggle to carve himself a personal imaginary home to express his creativity as a sublimation of his sense of alienation and exile.[4]

In this chapter, the tetralogy's actual text will 'speak' for itself, laying bare the author's reflective process. As Anäis Nin, Durrell's friend, wrote:

> What then should the critic do? Where should he look for his criteria? Inside the work itself, its universe and its mythology. He must look at it, listen to it, and simply say whether it is true to its own nature. The best judgment is a careful exposition of the work itself. For that, the work must be allowed to speak, uncoloured by preconception or prejudice.[5]

The interpretation of the text will rely upon particular images and phrases which represent the conscious and unconscious effort made by the author to explore his subjective experiences in the quest for the primeval experience of belonging to a homeland.

Three perspectives will be employed, each using the tension between the biographical and fictional elements of the work.

The first perspective views the city as a cradle where one aspires to realise and give form to one's unique voice. The city in this context appears to be a relatively neutral base, a mere backdrop against which the protagonist's escapades are set. In this context, the protagonist does not place any particular emphasis on the connection between himself and the city, nor is the city itself particularly significant.

The second perspective, evident mostly through his letter correspondence during those years, is Durrell's experience of Alexandria as a very significant and historically specific location of unique resonance, where he resided between 1941 and 1945 and met his second wife.[6] His time in the city was a stage in his world travels, as he was moving from one residence to another, only to find peace in none. Those were his years in exile, starting from his departure from India at the age of eleven and concluding at the age of forty-five, when he settled in the south of France. The interpretation of the letters is equivalent to the interpretation of prose when it comes to the tension between the biographical and fictional elements. Therefore, reading and interpreting the letters actually written at that time does not amount to finding hard evidence of Durrell's actual experiences which were then turned into prose in his later writing. Letters are as real, or not, as fiction, in relation to truth. Reading letters, like reading prose, permits yet another glance into the reflective processes Durrell was involved in during that time.

The third perspective treats Alexandria as the central protagonist in the tetralogy. The city takes an active role in forming the relation between the individual and his place of residence.[7] It becomes the liminal space where the individual experiences his highest and lowest moments. The city is the seed that sprouts his personality, the echo and shadow of his primal experience, which he aspires to restore and return to as a lost and forbidden Eden. The city of Alexandria stands as evidence of the author's reflective quest for meaning in life.

The topographic return to Alexandria

The return to the city in *The Alexandria Quartet*, as an *imaginary return* to the lost homeland, will be portrayed in light of the French philosopher Gaston Bachelard's (1884–1962) notion of *reverberation*. Bachelard wrote of the ways the city transforms the understanding of the individual of his self and the society that he inhabits. Alexandria, one of Durrell's many residences where he felt not-at-home, is at once a concrete place as well as a psychic enclave that functions as a safe haven from threatening external circumstances, a symbolic space where the internal workings of the mind, shown by dreams and poetry, take place. The external world does not cease to affect the individual – rather, the activities of the outside world and the impressions of the inner world echo one another.[8] *Reverberation* describes the relation between the actual event taking place in the external world and its *reverberated* impression that appears in the unconscious part of the self. The City is therefore not merely a description of the landscape or environment designed to set the narrative and characters against a certain backdrop. It constitutes an emotional element that is as significant as the narrative or characters. The actual experience of the city becomes an experience that offers *a poetic space* for the author. In his writing, the author returns in his mind to the city that he has internalised as an array of inner images that constitute his reflective process. How does that *imaginary return* happen?

The idea that external reality is registered and reflected in the mind of the individual is a fairly basic concept in psychoanalysis.[9] The British psychoanalyst Christopher Bollas refers to that process as *the topographic return*. In his book *Forces of Destiny*, Bollas describes the process that sees psychic experiences submerged in the unconscious and re-emerge later in the form of transformed psychic events as *the topographic return*.[10] He tries to describe the actual path taken as our sensual experiences are translated and transformed into psychic impressions (*internal objects*) over time, as well as into recurring intersubjective and behavioural patterns.[11] Bollas emphasises the significance of the time factor required for primal and formative experiences to evolve into *internal objects* that later generate contact with the external environment through language, art and interpersonal communication. He charts the process whereby sensory experiences translate into *internal objects* and then is represented through symbolical expression by using a series of six stages that form *the topographic return*:

1 Having an actual sensory experience (the actual *object*).
2 Creation of an internal mental space for digesting that experience.
3 A psychic representation of the internal *object* is formed in that mental space.
4 The internal *object* affects the way new actual sensory experience is digested.
5 Holding of the internal *object* allows the individual to be in reality and use the actual *object* without anxiety.
6 The actual *object* is now a subjective *object*, i.e. part of the personality of the individual.

The writing of the *Quartet* is such a *topographic return*. The experiences Durrell had in Alexandria in the 1940s (*the actual object*), integrated into his earlier experiences (*psychic representation*) after he had left (*mental space*), were transformed (*instincts*) on their way to becoming the raw material for *The Alexandria Quartet* (*holding of the internal object*) and allowed the writing of the novel. All the sensorial experiences he recounts in his letters were internalised by him and brought out in his writing, moulded also by his life circumstances in the years of working on the *Quartet*. The actual phenomenon of Alexandria was internalised by Durrell, underwent intrapsychic processing in his mind during the intervening years and acquired its symbolical representation with the literary object of *Alexandria* as featured in the *Quartet*. The *topographic return* is at once a return to the place itself, and a return to those unconscious primary experiences in his life.

The actual city of which Durrell wrote is nowhere, and never was, to be found in reality. Ironically, the institutions of the City of Alexandria formally commemorated the *Quartet* and a permanent exhibition of Durrell and his oeuvre is on display in the Alexandria library. Durrell himself received angry letters from readers who had taken the trip to Alexandria only to find it was nothing like his portrayals of it.[12] Even early studies of the *Quartet*, like the one written by Herbert Howarth in 1972, have argued that Durrell's Alexandria is the city he had read about rather than the city in which he resided during the war.[13] Howarth claims that Durrell's portrayal of the city's quarters, its people and the events that took place in it, is evidence that his impression of the city was mostly literary. He further claims that Durrell had not based his novel upon his own personal impressions of the city, but rather used other texts written about it as a source of inspiration. Howarth quotes E. M. Forster's (1879–1970) book *Alexandria, a History and a Guide*, published in 1922, as one such inspiration, alongside roughly a dozen other references, some of which were found in Durrell's library. Mona Morcos found many inaccurate concrete particulars in Durrell's portrayal of the city to prove that any relation between the actual city and the one created by Durrell as a fictional space was virtually accidental.[14] Contrary to Durrell's assertion in the prefatory notes to *Justine* that only the city was real, the city is perhaps the single most fictional element of the entire work.

In the preface to the new edition of *The Alexandria Quartet*, issued to mark the author's centenary, Jan Morris writes that the *Quartet* belongs to the genre of place-based novels, and should thus be seen in the context of his repeated attempts to find himself a place he could call home.[15] Between 1935 and 1980, Durrell wrote more than a dozen books that described his stay in different cities and countries, which should be thought of as *foreign residence books*.[16] Morris's treatment of Durrell's Alexandria as yet another city in a series of cities and countries in which he has resided echoes the ambivalent reception of Durrell in recent years, but in my eye treats the subject with undue lightness. More favourable to Durrell's deliberate and perhaps unconscious effort, Evine Hashem sees Durrell's Alexandria as a link in a long chain of cities that many writers have chosen as the base for their protagonists' plots, acknowledging that the city in those cases is more than a backdrop and frame story.[17] In so doing, Hashem joins earlier critics like Carl Bode, who, already in 1961, viewed the city as the protagonist of the entire work, and offers further examples from the works of Henry James (1843–1916) and Charles Dickens (1812–1870).[18] The fate of the protagonists of the work is bound up with the history of the city. A city like Alexandria, or London, was chosen by the writer for its particular history and imaginary resources to evoke in the author and reader alike the treasures of associations strewn in its streets, building, parks and bars. Strolling through the streets of the city, as it is depicted in the book, is like strolling through the mind and soul of the protagonists.

Over the years, many attempts have been made to get to the bottom of Durrell's "real" attitude to Alexandria. Did his time spent in the city indeed shape his writing in a way that no other city could, or had he used Alexandria to express his ideas, without this city ever permeating his consciousness? Is the city indeed the tetralogy's protagonist or is it a mere vibrant, exotic backdrop to the tropes of the tormented main narrative voice and protagonist, Darley? It is not my intention to either confirm or refute the dynamic between the fictional and biographical elements in the author's attitude to Alexandria, but rather to show how their affinity reflected in his work in multiple – and at times contradictory – ways.[19] Alexandria served as a host to Durrell's life experiences by perhaps intentionally disregarding the border between biography and fiction, thus reflecting Durrell's general only-too-human ambivalence regarding borderlines, an ambivalence I believe that is shared by most writers and artists. Durrell used the city to express his experience of it in the 1940s, while enduring a complex personal crisis, including the impact of his forced exile from his beloved Greek island, followed by a gradual deterioration of his relationship with his first wife, Nancy Isobel Myers (1912–1983), until the complete failure of their marriage. These crashing experiences are Durrell's formative experiences in writing the *Quartet*. Writing this work allowed Durrell to process these events as part of his exilic experience. Having completed the work, Durrell experienced a mental and spiritual recovery that allowed him, among other things, to eventually settle in the south of France, where he spent more than three decades, until his death. In the following pages, I will explore all three perspectives outlined earlier regarding the role and place that Alexandria had in Durrell's world. The three perspectives do not attempt to form a single all-inclusive analysis but rather offer a wide and endless horizon of interpretation which can also be contradictory at times.

The author, *the Heraldic Universe* and loneliness

The core of the first perspective is Durrell's *raison d'être*, as he stated time and again throughout his life – the only creative channel open for the artist to confer meaning on his life is through finding his own singular, solitary voice. In this perspective, Alexandria seems to have formed a mere vibrant backdrop to the existential dilemmas facing man. The "right" attitude to life dictates indifference and scepticism towards what goes on in the world, as it exerts no significant influence over our life and creative powers. The road to self-fulfilment is oblivious to political reality and historical context. The nature of the country's regime is a secondary, ephemeral fact for him and does not leave a mark on the personal struggle. This view incubated in Durrell during the 1940s, while living in Egypt. From these years on, as Ian S. MacNiven (born 1938), Durrell's friend and biographer writes, Durrell lost any interest in the political and public life and believed the only path to any change was through a shift in one's consciousness, even though the time he spent in Cyprus and Belgrade taught him a lesson about the raw realities of local politics.[20] This tunnel-view observation, which overlooks social and cultural contexts and deems individualism an end in itself, is well articulated in his 1938 letter to Miller: "The foundation is being quietly laid. I AM SLOWLY BUT VERY CAREFULLY AND WITHOUT ANY CONSCIOUS THOUGHT DESTROYING TIME."[21] What is this *destroying time* that Durrell pronounces as his goal? It is his effort to elevate the individual into a position where he can succeed in his quest beyond the bounds set by mortality. The quest of the individual for self-discovery needs to happen regardless of the limits that the passage of time imposes. Thus, Alexandria as a real city is less relevant; it is significant only as a backdrop and outer shell for his inner experience.

In his preface to the 1962 edition, Durrell challenged the contemporary notion adopted by modern literature concerning linear time, stating that he intended that the narrative story of his protagonist would not follow traditional concepts of sequential time perception.[22] The four volumes have to be read as a word continuum, not based upon time. As I wrote in the second chapter, he proposed that the first three volumes would be siblings, belonging to the same family and not necessarily following one another as sequels. Only the last volume he intended to be the only real sequel and continue the flow of narrative time. The work as a whole would challenge what is considered to be conventional in contemporary literature. Durrell defied the domination of the contemporary chronological narrative which was the leading literary norm. He challenged the inherent historical nature of the novel. No longer significant, the course of time relegates to the margins the historical and cultural circumstances that attend the events, at least temporarily. In order to follow the evolution of the inner world of the protagonist, chronological time must be stayed to make way for another perception of reality.

This perception places great emphasis on the inner world of the protagonists as the meta-structure of the whole novel, even once the individual is discovered to be overpowered by greater external forces, as I have explored in chapter three. The inner world of the individual has to be guarded and isolated so as not to be disturbed. This endeavour is referred to by Durrell as *the Heraldic Universe*. This world becomes a world marked by existential loneliness where his instincts and creativity have no boundaries. The solitude of the creative individual, focusing on his inner world, results in the somewhat patronising attitude he adopts towards his surroundings, perceiving the world he lives in as an opposition to his creative urge. *The Heraldic Universe* is a key concept in Lawrence Durrell's *Weltanschauung*. He first employed it in his seminal letter from August 1936 to his mentor, Henry Miller, where the two discussed their disagreement with the Surrealist movement and its emphasis on social change, which Durrell rejected:

> Listen, Miller, what I feel about it is this. To have art you've first got to have a big personality, pass it through the social mincer, get it ready for misery. Art nowadays is going to be real art, as before the flood. IT IS GOING TO BE PROPHECY, in the biblical sense. What I propose to do, with all dead solemnity, is to create my Heraldic Universe quite alone.[23]

Durrell declares his intention to set out on a journey that will establish his identity as an artist. This journey is going to take place through his writing whereby he will establish *the Heraldic Universe*. He describes it as the journey of the creative man, who is inevitably a lonely man. In this statement, Durrell binds together his psychological development and the creative process of writing. He refers to *the flood* as a formative experience that he will try to recover from. What he will attempt to do, he writes to Miller, is to return to a primeval state before humanity was punished by God for its wicked ways. Using such a mythological reference attests to the gravity with which Durrell viewed his efforts. It was not just a literary trick or gesture; it was his life's effort, the justification for his existence. Through his work, he will assume the position of *the prophet*, again a biblical reference, to correct his ways and lead the world towards a better future.

In a letter dated January 1937 to Miller he returns to *the Heraldic Universe* and tries to clarify what it means for him, adding the spiritual dimension to the duty of every artist to leave his mark and express in writing his unique inner world. "Now we have the timely recognition that each man is entitled to his own reality, interpret it as he wants. THE HERALDIC REALITY."[24] What did Durrell exactly mean by *the Heraldic Universe*? This has remained a point pondered by many Durrellians. Still its precise literary meaning has been left obscure, perhaps since it remained so, perhaps deliberately, in Durrell's own mind. Only towards the end of his life, he provided what might be seen as a clear definition. In his most autobiographical book, *A Smile in the Mind's Eye*, where he also revealed for the first time his agony following the death by cancer of his third and most beloved wife, Claude, he wrote:

> I note also the use of the adjective "heraldic" for which I have often had to answer the critics. It means simply the "mandala" of the poet or of the poem. It is the alchemical sigil or signature of the individual; what's left with the ego extracted. It is the pure nonentity of the entity for which the poem stands like an ideogram![25]

Perhaps a clearer definition would spoil the idiosyncratic charm the term holds. It is perhaps best to think of it as a poetic expression of what Durrell held most dear in his life. Like a poem, it is advised to allow its magic to work without taking it apart to examine its workings. Still, it might be safe to say that Durrell tried to signify the solitude of the individual and the ultimate value of self-expression as a value that cannot be surpassed. Durrell introduces *the Heraldic Universe* as a spiritual symbol of the individual aspiration for fulfilment and the realisation of his inner vision.[26] The vision he had was inspired by Taoist thought, particularly its Zen school. "His book (Lao Tzu and Chuang Tzu) had formed a sort of bond between me and my youthful preoccupations which had all got themselves crystallized around the notion of Tao . . . yet the awakening, pour ainsi dire,[27] was not just of a poetic order – though if I call it 'religious' I mean it rather in the anthropological sense and not in the denominational."[28] Durrell was influenced by the Taoist tradition at a young age, and refers to it in his seminal letter to Miller where he urged him to read different Zen scriptures as part of his scathing attack upon contemporary writers.[29] He first came upon Zen books in Corfu, before arriving to Paris in 1937, and it was the Taoist outlook that shaped his thought during those formative years.

Durrell viewed the formation of *the Heraldic Universe* as a cause worth committing himself to, almost as if he were establishing a new (this time chosen) homeland. *The Heraldic Universe* was his own exclusively and he intended to establish it as his private world, his real and true lost-and-refound homeland.

> But I tell you seriously that the heraldic universe when I get through with it, will be the only habitable place. It will be full of creators of real calibre . . . it will never be chic because it is my personal property and I don't want any movements made up of people who agree with each other even on first principles.[30]

This homemade homeland would never be in vogue and cannot be contained under any social, cultural, artistic or political movement. The world that Durrell speaks of is elitist, free of people who seek any kind of social alliance. Only artists who abide by Durrell's worldview will inhabit it. It will be a world where no disagreement could exist, as there is only one individual, a world where he holds complete control. He fancies himself in a homeland where he was the only man, with his voice the only one heard. In this kind of world, there is no room for the other, it is a world where the individual shoulders his solitude, the ghastly solitude, of the foreigner, the eleven-year-old boy sent away from home. Durrell's loneliness in his imaginary homeland is complete, or so he would like to believe, as he puts in the words of Clea, Darley's confidante and eventually lover, when she speaks of her solitude as not depriving her at all as she cannot be anyone other than who she is. She hints that the only failings she might have within her are invisible to the world. As the solitary being she is, love no longer has any value for her.[31] Through Clea, we can read between the lines that Durrell was indeed aware, though did not express it too openly, that "the fault" in his vision of *the Heraldic Universe* was the fact that in it, the artist would have his own shortcomings to contend with. These might be harder to deal with than any other person or relationship.

The solitude that Durrell preaches as a prerequisite for real creativity and freedom reflects a popular conviction of the period. Social psychologist Anthony Storr (1920–2001), for example, argues in his 1988 book *Solitude* that the emphasis placed by modern psychological theories on the importance of social relationships as a key for mental health and creativity is too great. He criticises what he views as the central psychological insight of the twentieth century, where the well-being of the individual is invested in the quality of their relationships. Storr says that the importance of relationships in the formation of the individual self should be considered alongside another, no less significant, factor, which is the creative activity that the individual is involved in.

> However important personal relationships may be for the creatively gifted person, it is often the case that his particular field of endeavour is still more important. The meaning of his life is constituted less by his personal relationships than by his work.[32]

He claimed that when the writer enjoys success, the attention his readers pay him is because of his work rather than his relationships. He further adds that even if the personal life of the writer is marred by fraught relationships with his family, for example, his success and potency will not rest exclusively on this element, but on the merit of their work. Such an argument is particularly pertinent to the case of the waning of public and critical attention to the works of Durrell after his death and after the revelations of his complex and sometimes abusive relationships with his family, wives and children. Yet this argument made by Storr, though perhaps not totally justified in perspective, is consistent with the outlook of Durrell himself as reflected in the term *the Heraldic Universe*. Durrell was willing to pay any social, personal or domestic price so as to have his vision reflected in his work. Individualism was his principle, guiding him throughout his life. His focus on himself paved the road for creating his inner world, in a manner that would guide him through life. The writing process was his golden road towards the promised land of literature, his own-made, imaginary homeland, even if he had to sacrifice his personal and marital happiness for it. As Pursewarden, one of the narrative voices of the *Quartet*, has written in his suicide letter-testimony to Darley, anyone who is able to transcend the gap that separates the world from *the Heraldic Universe*, discovers that he also has to make the rules for his conduct in it.[33]

Durrell's wish to establish his inner world through the process of overcoming pain, as expressed in his letter to Miller, echoes ideas expressed by the German philosopher Friedrich Nietzsche (1844–1900).[34] As with Freud and his influence on him, Durrell tried to underplay the influence of others in shaping his writing and thus there is very little reference to Nietzsche in his work. Freud himself viewed Nietzsche as an inspiration for some of the concepts that later came to underpin psychoanalytic theory; he even regarded Nietzsche as the man who had engaged in self-study more than any other man.[35] The Freudian idea that the individual is controlled by unconscious urges appears in Nietzsche's writing decades before it was articulated by Freud.

> So we are necessarily strangers to ourselves, we do not comprehend ourselves, we have to misunderstand ourselves, for us the law "Each is furthest from himself" applies to all eternity – we are not "men of knowledge" with respect to ourselves.[36]

In his book *On the Genealogy of Morality*, published in 1887, Nietzsche wrote of the inner search and its part in establishing man's belonging to his homeland. Nietzsche pointed to the direction Durrell was to assume decades later, as he commenced working on the *Quartet* as part of the journey to establish his own identity. The suffering which forms part of the maturational process that the artist must undergo if he is to achieve the clarity required to constitute his inner world lies at the heart of Nietzsche's thought. In his book *Ecce Homo* (1888) Nietzsche wrote of the solitude required for the creative experience, the same solitude that provided the clarity of mind.

> Those who can breathe the air of my writings know that it is an air of the heights, a strong air. One must be made for it. Otherwise there is no small danger that one may catch cold in it. The ice is near, the solitude tremendous – but how calmly all things lie in the light! How freely one breathes! How much one feels beneath oneself![37]

At the opening of *Justine*, Darley writes that he has arrived at the island where he lives in solitude with his books, so as to heal and seek the kind of clarity described by Nietzsche. In order to achieve clarity of mind and deal with the core issues of existence, he must isolate himself from all the moral and cultural influences that bore upon his mind. It is only when he is left alone with his thoughts, away from culture and moral issues of right or wrong, that he can reach the depths of his soul.[38] His solitude reflects his wish to get away from the culture he feels bound and restricted by, so that he can apprehend it from the perspective he desires to allow himself the freedom he requires for his creative fulfilment. Paradoxically, the primal place of belonging is perceived as a place the individual has to be exiled from if the individual is to exist creatively, but also as a place that one aspires to return to. Nietzsche thought of this primeval place, the culture to which the artist belonged but tries to remain at a distance, as an experience that tamed the individual into a civilised and cowardly behaviour.

> Supposing that what is at any rate believed to be the "truth" really is true, and the meaning of all culture is the reduction of the beast of prey man to a tame and civilized animal, a domestic animal, then one would undoubtedly have to regard all those instincts of reaction and resentment through whose aid the noble races and their ideals were finally confounded and overthrown as the actual instruments of culture.[39]

It is the products of this culture that breed the disease described by Nietzsche as man's weakness. It is this weakness that renders him an inferior and fearful creature, forced to live in moral decadence. The road to recovery back to proud and virile humanity lies in overcoming his fear through the conditions afforded by solitude. "My Humanity is constant over-coming. But I need solitude – which is to say, recovery, return to myself, the breath of a free, light playful air."[40]

In *Justine*, Darley describes himself as being sick. It is only a sick person that would choose to remove himself from the world in order to heal.[41] Nietzsche warns that the individual must choose carefully his solitude in order to heal. The wrong choice will entrench him in his misery and drive him away from his goal. "A mistaken choice of place and climate can not only estrange a man from his task but can actually keep it from him: he never gets to see it."[42] Durrell chose Alexandria as the arena where he would face his perils and overcome them. Through the process of writing, he hopes to uncover within his "real" inner experience, his *Heraldic Universe*. As Nietzsche wrote, one can only extract from his experiences that which he already knows. "For what one lacks access to from experience one will have no ear."[43] Therefore, the quest for *the Heraldic Universe* is a spiritual quest. It was his life circumstances which exiled him from that place. Finding *the Heraldic Universe* amounts to unearthing the extant.

The choice Durrell made of Alexandria as the suitable arena for his liminal experience is not only because it allowed him to find that which he already knows. Rediscovering the deeply buried experience that eluded him due to the traumatic experience he has endured is one part of the picture. No less significant is the portrayal of the world as corrupt and mean. The city of Alexandria seems the perfect candidate. For Durrell, the Anglo-Indian white man, brought up in a privileged and puritan British colonial atmosphere, the city of Alexandria with its 1930s–1940s concoction of cosmopolitan and oriental flavours formed an enticing stage. In order to accomplish his goal, Durrell describes Alexandria as an overpowering entity and invests it with magical powers. It is the city that controls the life of its inhabitants, it decides their destiny. It is only through extreme inner effort that the individual can resist and overcome the malevolent and decrepit city and instate his personal destiny in it. The struggle of the individual in the city is a struggle against dark, magical forces that signify the individual's deepest and most-feared, untameable and wild sexuality.

The notion of the city as an entity that must be overcome in order to achieve the psychic catharsis required for creative life leads Durrell to assume an aloof position that treats the Orient as a container for all that he disavows in himself. The existential solitude that Durrell called for allows the writer to elaborate his inner world, as reflected in *the Heraldic Universe* concept. Thus he can reach the high realms he aspired to, but at the price of splitting off and projecting unwanted aspects of his personality onto the world outside. In psychoanalytic theory, the process whereby the individual attributes to others unrecognised and unwanted aspects of himself is termed *projective identification*.[44] It is possible to see how Durrell's aloofness and detachment are accompanied by the aura of exoticism he attached to the Orient in general and to Alexandria in particular. Anne Zahlan notes how Durrell portrays Alexandria as a remote, unattainable city where exotic events take place, making it hard for the reader to experience and identify with them. The city of Alexandria is described in the novel not as an actual mundane place people live in. It is rather seen as an idealised or devalued portrait of a private fictional version of a city. It might even be another city, rather than a unique geographical and historical location inhabited by actual people, not just by the author's figments of imagination.[45] One could argue that the need and choice of a remote geographical platform to contain specific personal existential experiences is no coincidence. Durrell could have chosen to set the plot of the *Quartet* in any city around the world. Darley's experience, so it seems, would not have lost validity in London, Athens, Paris or any other city which Durrell knew and in which he resided before writing *The Alexandria Quartet.* Was Alexandria chosen because it is located in the East and unconsciously representing the oriental Other for Durrell, who himself belongs to the Imperial ruling class? If so, Durrell is of course not the first white Western writer to use the Orient for his projection of accounts of existential experiences which seem to disagree or be in disharmony with his sense of self. As Roland Barthes wrote in his book *Mythologies:*

> All told, exoticism here shows well its fundamental justification, which is to deny any identification by History. By appending to Eastern realities a few positive signs which mean "native," one reliably immunizes them against any responsible content. A little "situating," as superficial as possible, supplies the necessary alibi and exempts one from accounting for the situation in depth. Faced with anything foreign, the Established Order knows only two types of behaviour, which are both mutilating: either to acknowledge it as a Punch and Judy show, or to defuse it as a pure reflection of the West.[46]

Durrell himself was familiar with the East-West colonial tension, which made Alexandria a potent and perhaps inevitable choice. As a white man born and raised in colonial India, leaving the sub-continent though he had at a young age, he returned to the East – to the British-ruled Alexandria, which was perhaps for him, a watered down version of some of the flavours of the sub-continent. In his thorough biography, MacNiven stresses the difficulty Durrell experienced in his contact with the local Egyptian population. While in Egypt, Durrell tried to avoid the local population as much as possible and integrated himself with specific social circles, particularly the European refugees flooding the city, and the Coptic and Jewish communities.[47] The overwhelming majority of the local Muslim population remained a distant crowd for him, with whom he held no dealings bar the minimum entailed by the coloniser-colonised relations dictated by the hegemonic model of the colonialist age. As Marquis Deep wrote in a study comparing Durrell and the Egyptian writer Naguib Mahfouz (1911–2006), Durrell writes of the Orient in a manner that is typical of colonialist writing.[48] The Orient as a dangerous *internal object* is polarised with his Western inner world. It is a place of darkness, of harrowing voices, inhabited by humans of lesser spirit, the beasts and the wild. Durrell is careful, though, and attributes the words of derision to Nessim Hosnani, an Egyptian Copt, himself belonging to a small community at odds with the Muslim majority, when he speaks of Africa, which is mistakenly seen by some as an extension of Europe, often finds its way to assert itself as quite different. According to Nessim, Africa is a continent of alarming darkness, where the wild cries of the animals are followed by the voices of subhuman men.[49]

When writing of the Orient, Durrell wrote from within the colonial paradigm. He populated his Orient with *internal objects* that felt foreign and threatening to the integrity of his world. As Diana Festa-McCormick wrote in 1979, the city that Durrell wrote about through his projections had become a whore in his eyes.[50] The city's portrayal as a beehive teeming with perverse sexual activities reflected his worldview of the Orient as an exotic location infested with forbidden sexual desires. As Balthazar reflects while commenting on Darley's manuscript, the European notion of love, for instance, is not relevant in the world of the Arab who is still living in a much simpler peasant-like manner. The psyche of the European man is tormented in a way that the simple Arab is not able to fathom.[51] Alexandria is the receptacle of all that Western enlightenment will not tolerate, like child prostitution, rape or incest, to cite but some, thus preserving the notion that white European culture is morally superior. Durrell reinforces the hegemonic power relations typical of the Imperialist era and reveals his Orientalist attitudes to Alexandria in general, particularly to its Arab inhabitants. Whether portraying them in a romantic or perverse manner, the cultural bias that informed Durrell's experience of the Arabs he lived among is plain to see. The Arab individual, according to the author, is a simplistic, shallow character. The psyche of the Arab is not tormented or split in the romantic manner that alienates him from himself and culture as is the more culturally advanced European. He is unsophisticated in the manner reserved only to the European. The inevitable tension that binds the colonisers and colonised cultures alike has been widely discussed in postcolonial studies.

As it is not within the scope of this study to fully explore the field, I will focus on one particular aspect. While the Indian-American sociologist Homi Bhabha claimed that this tension had created a single colonialist subject,[52] the Kenyan-American Abdul R. JanMohamed (born 1945) argues that such an interpretation attests to an interpretive naivety and misses the point, which is the clear, unequivocal intention that the coloniser has in mind for the colonised.[53] The nature of this intention, which exemplifies the actual political power relations, can be revealed when we look into the actions of the colonisers, rather than examining their explanations or motives. These power relations are permanent and constant and are visible in any aspect of life. The racial differences between the colonisers and colonised create patterns of behaviour that saturate the language of the colonisers and colonised. Furthermore, the very notion of racial differences and the linguistic implications are moulded by the current power relations. Even writers who are aware of these power relations and oppose them are inevitably subjected to their sway and to the conditions produced by them in language and reality. JanMohamed differentiates between two colonialist stages. The first, dominant stage takes place during the early years of the colonisation, when the local culture is under the foreign culture's yoke. This stage comes to an end when the ruling culture "grants" the locals independence, yet maintains its presence by forcing forms of government and political practices on the newly independent political entity. It is this second, hegemonic stage that marked the cultural setting of Durrell's childhood in Anglo-India, and it is its values that he internalised and applied, consciously and unconsciously, when writing on Alexandria and the other places he lived in over the years.

The 1941–1945 correspondence

In order to illustrate how the dominant narrative voice of *The Alexandria Quartet* evolved out of the cultural context of 1940s Alexandria, the following pages will offer an interpretation of Lawrence Durrell's correspondence during the period that he spent in Alexandria. In his correspondence with friends, Durrell described the complex experiences he had in Alexandria between 1941 and 1945. The most significant correspondence was the one he held with Henry Miller, who spent those years travelling around the United States of America in his own quest.[54] This correspondence offers a rich vein of information that sheds light on the impression left by Alexandria on Durrell. Those years etched a deep mark in Durrell's consciousness, which transpired about ten years after leaving Alexandria, when he started working on the *Quartet* while living in Cyprus. Durrell arrived at Alexandria from Greece and through Crete in 1941, aged twenty-nine, with his first wife Nancy and their young daughter. It was a dramatic sail across the Mediterranean, dogged by the German Luftwaffe airstrikes at the Cretan port of Chania and upon disembarking in Alexandria. His departure from Crete was hasty, as he greatly feared for his own safety and the safety of the family. Durrell left behind many valuables, including manuscripts that would consequently be lost.[55]

He wrote of this experience in the *Quartet*'s fourth volume, when describing Darley's return to Alexandria. The airstrikes left their mark on him. Durrell's rich poetic language when describing the airstrikes only thinly disguises the anxiety encapsulated by this experience and the sense that his literary return to Alexandria means returning to a world that is not reduced to rubble just yet, but soon will be. It is a return to disaster, to witness the ruin of the city. It is just not the city itself that is ruined. The real ruin lies in the destruction of *the city* as the author remembered it. He returns there only to realise his memory is no longer intact. He goes back to a city that is no longer the same liminal space in which he struggled to reform his sense of the lost primeval home. He returns to the city to bear witness to the demise of the person he was. In those passages that describe his return, he writes about the terrible moaning sound that reminded him of the wings of an ancient and frightening bird. It was in fact the sound of the sirens, warning of a forthcoming shelling, but it sounded like the cries of souls caught in limbo. As they approach the coast, he sees in the sky the columns of smoke created by the rising rockets. They remind him of a huge ugly spider, suspended in the skies, leaving behind clusters of colourful explosions. The air above and the water below seem to be shaking with the terrible sounds and sights of the bombing. It is a moving apocalyptic description of the city as it seems to crumble right in front of his eyes.[56]

Durrell's departure from Greece following the imminent advent of the Nazi forces interrupted a relatively good period in his life. It seemed as though Greece had become for Durrell an adopted home and provided him with his kind of geographical and cultural climate, the closest to the India experience of homeland. In a conversation with Peter Adam, Durrell referred to Greece as his second place of birth.[57] Durrell's escape to Egypt and his forced stay there was a repetition of his sense of exile. He had hoped that having found Greece meant that his exile days were over. Alas, Egypt was the first stop in a series of cities and countries along Durrell's migratory trail between 1941 and 1958, when he settled in the south of France, where he rediscovered resonations of the belonging experience he had felt back in Greece. Southern France was his home until his death thirty-two years later.

Second World War Alexandria was altogether different than it appears today. Its proximity to Europe and comparative accessibility made it a relatively comfortable destination for many European nationals who had fled the advancing Germans and Italians. Alongside Durrell, thousands of refugees arrived at Alexandria, many of whom, like him, were intellectuals and men of letters.[58] The local population was a unique mix of religions, nations, languages and cultures, rendering Alexandria a cosmopolitan city that integrated Greek, Roman, Christian, Jewish and European cultural elements, in a rich tapestry that was nevertheless Egyptian by essence. The tension between the Muslim majority and Coptic minority bred intrigues and attempts by each group to overcome the other, at times by striking pacts with the ruling Imperialist power. This tension seems to have yielded one of Durrell's inspirations for the idea that informs the *Quartet*'s political plot, the Coptic scheme to join arms with the 1930s Jewish underground in Palestine so as to stamp out a possible political alliance between the Egyptian Muslim Mufti and the British Ambassador.[59]

Since its foundation in 332 BC by Alexander the Great, Alexandria formed a cultural hub of the Greek, Roman and Ottoman empires, with each conquering power stamping it with its architectural, social and cultural mark. The 1882 British conquest introduced a new governing structure to Egypt at large and particularly to Alexandria, where the local government was left in place, under British supervision and control.[60] The city's diverse population was a human mosaic brought to life thanks to its interaction with the surge of European refugee population in the 1930s–1940s.[61] For Durrell, according to his letters from the period, this was at once a vibrant literary setting, where he co-published a literary magazine with several other refugee writers and poets, which also served as a platform for his poems. It was also a setting where he found new sexual horizons in the intervening period between the collapse of his first marriage and his second marriage. In his months as a newly divorced man, Durrell plunged into Alexandria's nightlife scene, which was later elaborately portrayed in the *Quartet*. The European refugees and the foreign currency they brought along boosted the city's nightlife as well as its prostitution. Durrell gave many accounts of his relevant experiences in his letters from the period and in the *Quartet* itself. "It's funny the way you get woman after woman: and exactly what it adds up to I don't know: each more superficial than the last Gaby, Simone, Arlette, Dawn, Penelope."[62] Both his biographers agree that his sexual experiences of that period left him with a deep, perhaps even traumatic, mark, whose traces can be gleaned between the pages of the *Quartet*.[63] Durrell's marriage to Nancy was foundering when they had arrived in Egypt. A little more than a year after arriving in Egypt, Nancy left with their daughter Penelope and moved to Jerusalem. This was meant as a temporary parting to ensure the safety of the two and keep them away from the German bombing and the German forces edging towards Egypt. Having arrived in Jerusalem, Nancy wrote a letter to Durrell, informing that she had no intention of returning. Even though he was aware of their marital difficulties, this was a blow for Durrell. Beyond the loss he felt over his wife's leaving, Durrell agonised over the forced separation from his daughter. He felt this parting to be a betrayal on the part of Nancy, while the disappearance of Penelope from his life was experienced as death. This motif was to crop up years later in the *Quartet*. One of the sub-plots of the novel concerns the daughter of Justine, who has mysteriously disappeared and preoccupies Justine and people around her for a long time, until the grim truth of her death transpires.

Durrell did not stay lonely for long. Having made attempts to make amends with Nancy, through long-distance efforts as well as a brief visit to Palestine that was facilitated by his work in the British administration, Durrell embraced hedonism. He continued doing so until he met Eve (Yvette) Cohen, who was to become his second wife and the mother of his second daughter, Sappho. Eve was an Alexandrian Jew, the daughter of a Tunisian coffee shop owner father and a mother of Turkish descent. A journalist by profession, she impressed Durrell deeply. The Oriental figure she cut, which struck Durrell as exotic and mysterious and was later to enchant him even further due to her complex life story, formed the basis for the character of Justine.[64] Durrell's falling in love with Alexandrian Eve, the exotic Jewess, the mystery woman, formed the first stage in Alexandria becoming part of his *unheimliche* experience in the search for the homeland he tried to return to in his writing. He wrote to Miller at the time, for example, telling him that, paradoxically, Eve was at once a familiar and alienated experience for him, during the emotional turmoil of breaking up with Nancy.

> She is the only person I have been able to talk to really; we share a kind of refugee life. . . . [I]t has been incredible to find a woman whose sex responses start upwards from the soles of her feet – without any corrupting romantic Anglo-Saxon nonsense.[65]

Alongside the joy and excitement that accompanied the new relationship with Eve and especially before that, Durrell wrote in his letters of painful experiences that paralysed his writing. He thought nothing of venting his frustration on the local population, which he described in very pejorative terms. In a 1942 letter to his friend, the poet Anne Ridler (1912–2001), he writes of the impasse he felt in Egypt: "I haven't felt like writing a line to anyone, being so dead to the world in this copper-pan of a blazing town with its pullulating stinking inhabitants."[66] Several months later, in a letter to Henry Miller from December 1943, having moved to Alexandria from Cairo, he writes of the inner death experience that grips him after Nancy had left him and moved to Jerusalem: "We are all so worm eaten by the war that I do not work at all. . . . We are dying steadily inside and hoping for it all to end as soon as possible."[67] He is unable to write. His stay in the city is only temporary for him and he hopes to be freed of it soon. He also writes longingly about Greece and the war, about being a refugee: "Greece is going right under this winter: heart breaking situation, famine, disease, and internal anarchy – walking murder abroad."[68] In February 1944, he writes again to Miller, he ventures to express some hope: "I have been so long barren that I fear to tell you that I am working once more: for fear I shall blow up and fall into an Alexandrian frenzy of apathy."[69] Durrell portrays his sordid experience in Alexandria in very vivid colours. Even when he writes that his creative power and his *joie de vivre* have been compromised, he is still able to write quite moving prose:

> The Alexandrian way of death is very Proustian and slow; a decomposition in greys and greens – by the hashish pipe or boys. But the women are splendid – like neglected gardens – rich, silk-and-olive complexions, slanting black eyes and soft adze-cut lips, and heavenly figures like line-drawings by a sexual Matisse. I am up to my ears in them – if I must be a little literal . . . but one has never had anything lovelier and emptier than an Alexandrian girl. Their very emptiness is a caress. Imagine making love to a vacuum. . . . When they make love, it's like two people in a dark room slashing at each other with razors – to make each other feel?[70]

The mixture between his psychic pain and the sensual whirlwind he indulges perhaps attests to the turbulent state he was in, and perhaps also to the impression he wished to convey to his mentor, Miller. But what he feels is genuine. He is truly confused and in pain as a letter written in March 1944 addressed to Diana Gould Menuhin (1912–2003), Yehudi's Menuhin (1916–1999) spouse, shows:

> Wonder how soon we can get out of this country. . . . Meanwhile the ubiquitous dust and blackness; the faces of the Arabs with their weakness and cupidity. The thin exhausted lusts of the Alexandrians running out like sawdust out of dummies; the shrill ululations of the black women, the rending of hair and clothes in mourning – a skilled occupation – outside the whitewashed hospital. The tarbush, the dark suit, the rings, the French accent; the scrofula, the pox, the riches, the food. Even in your Italian brothel I cannot think how to write or speak to you from this flesh-pot, sink-pot, melting-pot of dullness.[71]

Durrell continues narrating his negative experience in Alexandria a month later. In a letter dated April 1944, he writes beautiful prose to Miller about his inner anguish in a world plagued by war:

> Middle East is a dead centre – the outer ring of the whirlpool moving slowly round and round – so we are all in limbo and deader than the really dead or the practically dying. . . . Everything is smashed up beyond words – internal economy, public services, currency. . . . I feel that the time is not ripe to reassert ourselves as artists and men yet. Anything we do is on the side until this great bloody farce is played out. I am writing a bit these days – very badly – like a man with a creeping paralysis.[72]

It would be absurd of course to claim that Durrell enjoyed the physical and emotional hardships of those days, but it is still plain to see from the abundant quotations brought here that his existential circumstances brought out some very precise and clear observations which he cherished and used later on in his writing of the *Quartet*. He feels no better even a month later, as emerges from his letter to Miller from May 1944. Despite his intimations of his life of debauchery, emotionally and spiritually his depression lingers, and Alexandria is portrayed unfavourably and repulsively, as a city crammed with lowly physical experiences that do not allow him any creative experience. Durrell describes the women and his sexual experiences with them in very derogatory words, degrading them in almost every possible sense. He is at his misogynist worst here. Greece is still cast as the idyllic, primeval haven from which he has been expelled and where he pictures himself returning. In the very same letter, he tells Miller that he had met Eve, the woman who will change his life and with whom he will undergo deep transformations, as will be described in the following pages and in chapter five.

> Here we are sweltering in an atmosphere that demands a toast – great passion, short lives. Everything is worn thin as an eggshell; it's the fifth year now and the nervous breakdown is coming out into the open. . . . The

> poetry I exude these days is dark green and streaky – like bad bacon. But the atmosphere of sex and death is staggering in its intensity. . . . Alexandria is, after Hollywood, fuller of beautiful women than any place else. Incomparably more beautiful than Athens or Paris; the mixture Coptic, Jewish, Syrian, Egyptian, Moroccan, Spanish gives you slant dark eyes, olive freckled skin, hawk-lips and noses, and a temperament like a bomb. Sexual provender of quality, but the atmosphere is damp, hysterical, sandy, with the wind off the desert fanning everything to mania. . . . No, if one could write a single line of anything that has a human smell to it here, one would be a genius. . . . I want a long rest from this incessant plucking of little people with little minds at the root of one's reason and self respect. . . . The next ten years should see us in full cry over the hills. . . . Simple needs this time. A girl who really fucks with the heart and soul and buttocks; an olive tree, a typewriter, and a few great friends like you.[73]

In an August 1944 letter to Miller, when the first signs of the imminent end of the war were showing, Durrell is in a position to conclude his exile experience in Alexandria.

> Now the war seems to have taken a definite turn and we hope that it will be over in a month or so. I am written down for Greece. I terribly need to recover my sanity a bit – disoriented and bruised a bit still, and haven't seen anything but sand and palms for two years. I did not know before what Gaul meant to the exiled Roman poet or Siberia to the Russian. Now I know. Your heart shrivels in its case for lack of moisture . . . one could not continue to live here without practicing a sort of death – hashish or boys or food.[74]

Durrell's thoughts are marked by fear of having been harmed by his hedonistic experiences and embracing Greece as the home he was exiled from and the place he hopes to return to. In March 1945, two months before leaving Alexandria on his way to Rhodes, Durrell writes to Miller again, describing the spiritual desolation he has experienced in Alexandria, his sense of ruin given the ravaging of the occupied continent, and his great hope that returning to Greece will breathe a new spirit in him.

> There is a horrid blank empty silence; the whole Middle East is a figurative and literal desert in which only the most awful literary blooms flower. . . . I have been like a prisoner writing on the wall with a rusty nail in order to keep sane. A little Aegean sunlight and freedom will give me the peace to undertake THE BOOK OF THE DEAD. It's all written in my head.[75]

Within this wasteland, a glimmer of hope twinkles, signalling that the end of the exile might be near as he already makes plans for his next book, the future *Alexandria Quartet*. At this point it was still *The Book of the Dead*, an apt name for his experiences of those years.

Durrell left Alexandria in spring 1945, having been posted by the Foreign Office to the island of Rhodes. When arriving at Alexandria in 1941, Durrell had been married to Nancy and by the time he left it in 1945 he was in a relationship with Eve. Though only four years, these were crucial for his formation as a writer. His stay in Alexandria, as demonstrated in the letters, was fraught with the crisis of his first marriage, as well as with creative aridity, a cultural experience of meagreness, his settling into a life of sexual debauchery and his encounter with a local population, which exposed his colonial roots. During those years, Durrell had a range of transformative experiences, with implications he was to process many years later through his work. As Gordon Bowker, the unofficial biographer of Durrell wrote:

> Durrell's Egyptian war was to transform him, for better and worse. The impact of Egypt and its strange mix of cultures, the unreal life lived by Europeans there during the war, the new literary friendships and tastes he developed, and the changes in his own personal circumstances, all helped to induce a ferment of ideas and a more exotic moral outlook than hitherto.[76]

The mark left by these experiences, as articulated in his letters, was internalised in him and would resurface later in *The Alexandria Quartet*. The years Durrell spent in Alexandria were his drought days, as they continued with his travels from one European country to another in his capacity in the British administration, as well as providing him with the raw matter on which he drew for his greatest inspiration when he commenced writing *The Alexandria Quartet*, the apex of his work. His exile from Greece brought back the sense of exile from India at the age of eleven. Alexandria provided him with the existential space to reckon again with his sense of alienation. For Durrell, his home is the place where he was not, the place he left and now misses and hopes to return to. In practice, Durrell cannot but fail to return to this imagined homeland. The return to the homeland is fictional. He can find some rest only through the act of writing which in turn preserves the paradoxical sense of *unheimliche* encountered deep within himself.

Alexandria as the mother-city

In the following pages I will walk through the city of Alexandria as it was created by the author of the *Quartet* as a liminal space. That space formed a psychic cloister, a place where his inner workings could be displayed. As Darley ruminates in the opening passages of *Justine*, he thinks about Alexandria and considers his days there as spaces between dreams. The passage of time seemed erratic and he felt the world asked nothing of him but to merely survive.[77] As such, it was familiar and homely and yet strange and frightening. A place he knew, but not enough. He could only discover more if he allowed himself to recognise that which he had willingly forsaken. Nietzsche wrote that one can only learn from his experiences what he already knows.

> Ultimately, nobody can get more out of things, including books, than he already knows. For what one lacks access to from experience one will have

> no ear. Now let us imagine an extreme case: that a book speaks of nothing but events that lie altogether beyond the possibility of any frequent or even rare experience – that it is the first language for a new series of experience. In that case, simply nothing will be heard, but there will be the acoustic illusion that where nothing is heard, nothing is there.[78]

Becoming familiar with what is *unheimliche* and integrating it can occur only because it was also *Heimlich*. That which seemed to be dead is actually alive, that which seems to be alive is actually dead.

The *acoustic illusion*, that silence, denotes the unconscious parts of the mind of the author, particularly those parts in his sexuality that also stem from his earlier past experiences, which constituted his consciousness as a writer. In his mind, Darley tries to retrace his way back to the city, to the place of origin.[79] Durrell seeks to return to the primeval city, and to himself, via the memory he picturesquely describes as iron chain links, themselves heavy and cumbersome. The return is by means of associations, link by link. It is a return to the city and the time in which the temporary delusion of being a master of his fate played out. He wonders if the memories he has are real or figments of his imagination. The return feels forced. He wishes he could stop digging in his wounds. But he cannot stop.[80] Such a forced return can be described as the Freudian *return of the repressed*. According to psychoanalytic theory, unresolved unconscious conflicts and traumatic traces of experience will continuously seek to surface into consciousness through the thoughts, emotions and actions of the individual. This is due to the instinctual content they hold which must be discharged either through symptoms, dreams or insight. Such a relieving insight can be gained in many forms, one of which is psychotherapy but certainly not the only one. If such a relief does not occur, the individual, like Darley, finds himself returning to a place of pain, a place he had hoped he had been released from by his departure and yet he finds that it keeps coming back to him from the nether of his soul. No rational explanation can explain why this is happening. No longer can he understand why he must keep going back to the same places in order to keep observing himself and all that he has been through. Only through introspection he finds such an allusion to an insight.

In the opening words of *Balthazar*, he refers to Alexandria as the *poetic mother-city* which he sees and recalls in every memory he has of the people and places of the city. That illuminating term is almost hidden in his flow of associations and needs a careful attention to single it out for what it is. Darley returns to Alexandria and establishes it as a *maternal entity* that is not just a passive space to accommodate human plots, but a generative womb-space where life is begun and forms its initial encounters with the world. It is the *mother-city* that has given its inhabitants life. It is the city that breathed life into its struggles with its inhabitants. The city is the unconscious that dominates the activities of the people. It is the city that begets and sustains its inhabitants.

Durrell's definition of Alexandria as the unconscious *poetic mother-city* is the key to understanding his writing about the city. The city is a mother sustained by the practice of writing and recollection. As Bachelard wrote, the city is a poetic space that retains the passions of its inhabitants.[81] The author's attitude to the poetic city is ambivalent based on the inner *unheimliche* experience, composed both by proximity and distance, love and hate. His love is the love of an exile to his homeland, as Durrell speaks through the mouth of Narouz, Nessim's wild brother, who says that he had always rejected and felt passionate about Alexandria in equal measures, as only an exile can.[82] What is this love of the exile towards the mother-city? When describing Alexandria as a mother-city, the author encapsulates the deep complexity of the attitude of the individual towards his homeland, the place to which he belongs. Belonging evokes intense feelings of affinity that may constitute a primeval experience of security and harmony. But belonging also evokes a reversed experience, a wish to differentiate and distance oneself, so as to avoid assimilation in an experience that can blur one's boundaries and independence. In her 1991 book *Strangers to Ourselves*, dedicated to the experience of exile through psychoanalytic perspectives, Julia Kristeva wrote:

> As far back as his memory can reach, it is delightfully bruised: misunderstood by a loved and yet absentminded, discreet, or worried mother, the exile is a stranger to his mother. He does not call her, he asks nothing of her. . . . The foreigner, thus, has lost his mother.[83]

Durrell stages the city as the primeval maternal place he wished both to revisit and draw away from, and in the process realises the full complexity of this ambivalence, nourished by the deeply felt *unheimliche* sensation. As he tries to differentiate himself from the city, he discovers that it is internalised in him, part of his psyche, keeping him bound to it even as he tries to break away. Alexandria is a *mother-city* internal object from which he was exiled. The maternal object and homeland object are two aspects of the same inner psychical structure. His banishment from his homeland is like the untimely separation of the son from his mother. His effort to reinstate the city as an omnipotence, as he does throughout the *Quartet*, reflects his effort to reconnect with the lost omnipotent object of his mother.

In the beginning of *Justine*, the very beginning of the journey, Alexandria is described as the place the protagonist revisits in order to understand all that he has endured. His memories take him back to the city where he spent a short but immensely significant time, the city which turns the lives of its residents inside out, in every sense, the city that pretends to be a welcoming host to its people but before long plants in them a host of conflicts upsetting their personal lives, the all-devouring *mother-city* that uses them as the flora that it relies on for sustenance.[84] The conflicts that the individual experiences in the city may at first seem to be unique, but this is no more than illusion. The individual himself is insignificant. His identity and destiny is determined by unknown forces.

To illustrate that seminal point which is repeated throughout the *Quartet*, Durrell employs two images. The first is of the individual stranded on an island, and the second is the star Arcturus. This star, also known as "Guardian of the Bear," inspired many myths over the years and across different cultures. According to Greek mythology, this star was created in order to guard the constellations Ursa Major and Ursa Minor.[85] It is also cited in the Book of Job under the name *Ash*: "Which maketh the Bear (Arctus), Orion, and Pleiades"[86] and "or canst thou guide the Bear (Arcturus) with his sons?"[87]. The use of this image of Arcturus, the Guardian of the Bear, suggests that the author was spared a tragedy by being snatched from his birthplace and placed in a faraway place where he was safe from the fate that lay in store for him. In other words, the author describes his exile to the Greek island as salvation from what would have been his tragic fate had he stayed in Alexandria. Darley continues and quotes Justine, who reassures him that he, and the rest of the people he had met in Alexandria, were mere pawns in the play that the city enacted upon them. Replacing *the city* with the Freudian *unconscious*, echoes the similarities the outlook Ancient Greece shared with psychoanalysis as far as the control the individual has over his life is concerned. Be it the Gods, the Oedipal complex, the lure of the mother or the unconscious, the individual is but a pawn in the hands of greater powers. The fate that the individual attempts to escape, eventually to no avail, is the Oedipal fate. His exile was meant to guard him against his fate, but as man cannot escape his psyche, he is bound to have to face his destiny.

The destiny that *the city* brings is the death of individual self, the very opposite of what Durrell meant by *the Heraldic Universe*. It does not permit the individual to maintain his illusory sense of cohesion. Once the individual has become aware of his destiny in the city, its ordinary locations, like its port and streets, do not exist in the same matter-of-fact that they did before. Quotidian reality goes over and beyond the minds of the protagonists. Nothing exists but the chimeric space of the dream and the experience of the self under attack. The city itself assails the ability of the individual to pursue any single continuous existence. His own authenticity and sense of agency is challenged, as Balthazar suggests to Darley when he advises him that the story he is telling needs to be told in layers. The narrative would be of sliding doors, where glimpses of different truths would appear, sometimes complementing one another and at other times negating each other. That would be the only way to do justice to the true nature of the city.[88] Darley himself concludes in the last paragraphs of *Justine* that Alexandria is a capital of memory where the boundaries between reality and memory are blurred. Even the memories themselves are slowly transformed in the city until he can no longer be sure whether what he remembers did take place or was invented.[89]

Durrell, Freud, Fliess and bisexuality

When trying to answer the question he posed to himself regarding the real nature of the city, Darley is confused. He sees the city as a series of images describing all that is implied by the name Alexandria: dust-tormented streets, flies and beggars. When describing the city's people, he takes it a step further: the residents of Alexandria inhabit an existential realm between the flies and beggars. There are five races, five languages and a dozen creeds in the city. There is one essence that links them all: sexuality. But it is no ordinary sexuality. It is sexual provender that lies all over the city, overwhelming its residents with its variety and profusion. Such a variety does not make Alexandria a happy place. Sexuality in Alexandria is perverse and inwardly turning. It does not seek to make fruitful contact through a Hellenic celebration of the sensual body. It tears apart the body and uses it as a winepress uses grapes to produce wine – it crushes people. Anyone who survives the crushing force of the city is sick, alone and wounded. The survivors of the city, like himself and like Nessim Hosnani, whose voice narrates this reality, are deeply and mortally wounded in their sex.[90]

The centrality of sexuality in the *Quartet*, as the driving force which charges the city with its potency and liminal quality, first appears in the epigraph of the *Quartet*'s first volume, *Justine*. The epigraph quotes a brief extract of a letter Freud wrote to his friend and pupil, Wilhelm Fliess (1858–1928), in August 1899. Durrell does not cite to whom it was addressed nor when it was written. The epigraph is one of the pillars that support the structure of the entire work as a headline. With its laconic, pithy and ambiguous content, this epigraph is the first of many indications of the central role sexuality takes in the complexity of the relations portrayed in the work. The epigraph as it appears in *Justine* is as follows: "I am accustoming myself to the idea of regarding every sexual act as a process in which four persons are involved. We shall have a lot to discuss about that."[91] Reading the original letter reveals that Durrell quoted only a specific part of the letter and it is this fragmentary extract that leaves a vague impression. Without reading the whole letter, its full meaning remains unclear.

What Freud wrote in the original letter is his understanding of the bisexual nature of all people in their sexual development. Every man and woman contains within themselves male and female parts which interact with one another, thus forming *four persons*:

> The farther the work of the past year recedes, the more satisfied I become. But bisexuality! You are certainly right about it. I am accustoming myself to regarding every sexual act as a process in which four individuals are involved. We have a lot to discuss on this topic.[92]

Part of the ample correspondence shared by the two men during 1887–1904, the letter offer a reliable source on the evolution of Freud's ideas. The letters show Freud engaging in the most intimate exposure of his personal and professional experiences during the period when he composed his major works, like *Studies of Hysteria* (1893–1895), *The Interpretation of Dreams* (1900) and *A Fragment of an Analysis of a Case of Hysteria* (1901), which in fact marked the inception of psychoanalytic thought. The letters exchanged with Fliess revealed Freud more intimately and openly than in any other later correspondence. In those years, Fliess was closest to Freud as they began their respective medical careers.[93] In the full letter Freud writes of his fear of the censorship he will have to face once his book is out.

Nevertheless, it seems he does not allow censorship, real or imagined, to interfere with his flow of writing.

Durrell used only a fragment in his epigraph which omits its main object, bisexuality, and not just because of censorship.[94] While such an omission is understandable and even justifiable, given his wish to outwit the censorship mechanism that indeed operated at the time, it is not the only factor. It is true that Durrell's early work was not published without restrictions, but I suggest that he cut Freud's bisexuality statement not just because he feared censorship but as an expression of his own ambivalence towards the complex sexual experiences he had witnessed and participated in during his years in Alexandria. His omission of the open reference to bisexuality relates to what he tried to repress – his complex sexual experiences during his years in Alexandria, which made him think of himself as sick.[95] The inner censorship he applied suggests a psychic conflict. Establishing Alexandria, *the mother-city*, as a poetic space where the protagonist comes face to face with his passions and undergoes a liminal process, created a complex, ambivalent experience in him. His wish of finding salvation through sexuality aroused his fear lest he encounter forbidden parts of his sexuality in this quest, like bisexual wishes, whose pursuit could result in mental illness. At the opening of *Justine*, the protagonist writes that Alexandria is like a winepress from which all the wounded-in-sex characters emerge. The *Quartet*'s plot is shot through with descriptions of perverted sexual experiences, including child prostitution and incest, sexual ecstasy during pagan rituals and masturbation. The sum total of these experiences makes Alexandria a space where sexual experience engulfs the individual, almost as a rite of passage. The sexual experience is described as an ecstatic-religious experience, even when playing out in the debasing conditions of child prostitution, and it meets one of Victor Turner's (1920–1983) definitions of the blend of lowliness and sacredness characterising liminal phenomenon.[96]

Sexuality in this work is not some practice enjoyed by its participants, but part of a ceremonial or even ritual experience they undergo perhaps even somewhat reluctantly. The narrative in the *Quartet* often shows Alexandria as ritualistic arena for ceremonies that see their participants shed, or lose, the traces of their quotidian identity so as to undergo deep consciousness experience. Sexuality is a compulsive human practice, a language. Darley refers to sexuality as a language that needs to be learnt, a language that uses the body and the skin for its vocabulary.[97] As part of his individualistic worldview, the author consciously and deliberately situates the sexual experience as a formative experience in the development of the individual. Such a position triggers a defence mechanism within him. Sexual practice is not only the experience of the protagonists, but is ascribed to the nature of the city as a whole. Alexandria is the sexual melting pot that dispossesses its inhabitants of their bodies. Sexuality becomes a total, all-encompassing experience. Sexuality is the city's means of controlling its inhabitants. It grants them neither happiness nor acceptance of their existential circumstances. However, it confronts them with a notion of themselves that undermines the ontological security of their life and sends them on an existential quest.

When Alexandria is described as inundated with sexual provender, it implies that human sexuality is an organic matter that serves as livestock feed. The narrator is not appreciative of this sexuality that he encounters in the streets of Alexandria. It is an Oriental sexuality that wouldn't even allow the body indulge in the anarchism of the senses – the body itself is left scathed by the force of this sexuality. The Oriental sexuality, unlike its Hellenic counterpart, strips the body of itself, leaving it to succumb to its weakness. The *Quartet*'s characters are left scarred by their encounter with sexuality, as Darley writes of his encounter with Melissa, whom he finds wounded in her sex, like a bird who has flown into the water and is flapping her wings for dear life.[98] The melting pot of Alexandria wounds everybody. Even if sexuality in Alexandria leaves the characters with neither mutilations nor mental injuries, they are nevertheless left exhausted. In Alexandria, sexuality is an element that cannot be overlooked. It is the fundamental streak in everybody's lives. Darley does not mince his words on that matter; as far as he is concerned, it is the sexual exhaustion that is the core of what he thinks of as the Mediterranean narcissistic preoccupation, its disease.[99] Sexuality makes or breaks the individual. When the individual, particularly the woman, succeeds in establishing her sexuality in a compelling manner, that is, in a sluttish manner, she acquires a goddess status (Justine), but when this effort fails, her fate will be harsh (Melissa). The woman therefore can be either a harlot or a goddess. Her status is determined relative to how she exploits her sexuality.

Durrell does not allow any of the main female protagonists a particularly good path in the plot: Justine, Darley's lover, is portrayed as an adulterous nymphomaniac who uses the men who cross her path for her personal ends; Melissa, Darley's previous lover, who works as an erotic dancer, dies of cancer; while his friend-turned-lover, Clea, is a reclusive painter who loses her right hand in a diving accident. In fact, the entire *Quartet* offers not a single happy outcome for any of the female characters in their engagement with the world. The relationships they engage in end in tragedy, breakup or infidelity. The woman, as noted, is either a harlot or goddess. The narrative voice fails to see her as the complex being he views himself to be as a man.

Darley proclaims that Justine is the prototype of all women. She is more than just a particular woman but an incarnation of womanhood in society, a goddess.[100] Every woman is a variation of the theme she embodies. She stands for the fate of every woman in the eye of the man. As long as she remains teeming with passions that generate a magnetic field where man feels trapped, collision with her is inevitable. Any attempt to explain her based on one theory or another will provide only a temporary respite from her mysterious influence. Justine defies explanation. In fact, the only way to explain her is by obliterating her sexuality and humanity and turning her into a mythical character. Paradoxically, it is only as a goddess that she is scaled back to proportions that the man can accommodate. No longer is she a woman, but an archetypal character devoid of any subjective content or cultural context. Her elevation to goddess status allow ignoring her humanity and social context. She then exists as a magical power, like the city of Alexandria. As female sexuality, as conceived by men, holds the key to his destiny, the men in this work realise they depend on her and are therefore trapped. As Darley wonders towards the end of *Clea*, it is hard for men to decide whether she was a nymph, a vampire or a goddess. She could be any of those, or all of them altogether. She was all that men wanted her to be. She was written to fit what men wanted her to be.[101] The power men invested in her imaginary character, the internalised image of her, ruled their lives. Their sense of identity seemed to be in her hands. As Balthazar said to Darley after reading Arnauti's account in *Justine*, the fate of the man is like the fate of Roman Antony, who was seduced by the tragic character of Cleopatra to stay in Alexandria, a move which consigned him to exile, stripped him of all his titles and eventually led to the death of both lovers. Sexuality, which at first appears to offer salvation, is not just that. It also spells death and sickness. If the individual fails to, or cannot, understand his place in the world, as happens to Darley, he finds that the world, the *mother-city*, becomes a sickness for him, and may even prove fatal. The sickness which he attributes to female sexuality can only be reckoned with by making her to be either a harlot or a goddess. Female sexuality precipitates his downfall unless he succeeds in channelling it to his needs and thereby relegating the woman where she is inferior to him. If that happens, she finds herself without her sexuality and thus has nothing. As Clea writes to Darley in *Justine*, she found that once Justine was no longer seized and motivated by her passions as her aspirations were not met in the male dominated world, she became devoid of all her energy. Once her sexuality had been extinguished, she lost her purpose in life and became absent-minded and forlorn.[102] Without sexual passion, she has nothing. As sexuality is the driving force behind all human behaviour and motivation once that was taken from her, she became mortally sick.

Durrell, Groddeck, sexuality and death

Durrell's inspiration to engage with the relation between man's sexuality and man's health – and probably with the bisexual question, which he was ambivalent about – followed his reading of one of Freud's pupils, Georg Groddeck.[103] It was probably in 1944 that Durrell came upon Groddeck's writings, which he avidly reported to Henry Miller in a letter from Alexandria, where he also mentions the issue of censorship I referred to earlier.

> There is only political censorship, and as I am on the side of the angels I guess you can send me anything . . . I'm absolutely bowled over by Groddeck's The Book of It – it's simply terrific. I have written England to send you a copy – I know you'll want to keep it.[104]

What excited Durrell about Groddeck's thought and found its way into the *Quartet*, as also evident in his choice of epigraph from Freud's letter to Fliess, concerns humans as bisexual by nature.

> I maintain the position that everything human is dependent on this infinitely mysterious entity and I also persist in maintaining that nobody can fathom

> the depths of the It. . . . Another form of the It which is more accessible to me I want to call the dual nature of the It. All human life can be seen as simultaneously male and female, child and grownup.[105]

But unlike the normalising tone with which Groddeck relates to bisexuality, in *The Alexandria Quartet*, bisexuality in particular and sexuality in general reflected an environment that bred sickness. Perhaps the starkest expression of this outlook, which I have already pointed to, is the character of the father of Capodistria. Supposedly a minor figure, it is telling that he presents his perfect relationship with a woman as one that can be conducted with a full-size rubber model of a woman, and thus end years of agonising relationships with real women.[106] The rubber doll as substitute for the actual woman is only one "solution" offered for the sexual question in the *Quartet*. When the woman is perceived as a figure existing in a different frame of reference than man, there are further options of twisting her figure so that man can hold on to his dominant position. The woman who exudes sexuality constitutes a threat to male dominance and must therefore be relegated to a baser level. As Balthazar remarks to Darley, making love with someone who is inferior to oneself carries an added perverted sexual value thanks to the knowledge that through the sexual act they would be initiated to the deepest and lowest realm of passions.[107]

Another of Groddeck's ideas that struck a chord with Durrell concerned the mind and body as a single inseparable entity.[108] Groddeck developed a far-reaching theoretical approach based on his clinical experience.[109] "There is no such thing as a I, it is a lie, a misrepresentation to say: I think, I live. It ought to be: it thinks, it lives. It, i.e. the great mystery of the world. There is no I."[110] The main concept coined by Groddeck and inspiring Durrell's enthusiasm was *It*. This concept sought to replace the Freudian topography of the *I* (*ich*), which Groddeck deemed insufficient.[111] He found that *the It* offered a more apt representation of the mystery of human existence, without reducing it to a single human being. "I had become convinced that the distinction between body and mind is only verbal and not essential, that body and mind are one unit, that they contain an It, a force which lives us while we believe we are living."[112] As evidenced by the letters Freud exchanged with the Russian psychoanalyst Lou Andreas-Salomé (1861–1937), Groddeck was credited with the concept of the Id, even though his overall influence on the psychoanalytic movement was played down.[113] Nevertheless, Groddeck's idea that there no single *I*, or *self*, as a cohesive entity excited Durrell. If the *I* did not exist as a unitary cohesive entity, there was also no single truth that could be established, laying the base for the manifold aspects of the narrative as appears in the *Quartet*. Groddeck did not stop at claiming that the *I* did not exist as a single unit. For him, this concept develops into the idea that our lives are not controlled by a clear, cohesive experience of our self, but by greater powers, which we can only identify at a distance and even then, only through their action on us and our environment.[114] When Durrell invests the city of Alexandria with control over the lives of the protagonists, he in fact hints at Groddeck's interpretation of the workings of *the It*. Man cannot presume to have control over his life, but must acknowledge that he is subjected to greater powers, in this case, Alexandria.

Sexuality, as experienced by Darley in the *mother-city*, exists as a phenomenon belonging to the liminal state from which the individual needs to heal and evolve. The impact sexuality has upon the psyche of the individual places the city as a memory which remains haunting. Although Darley has experienced it as half imaginary, he has no doubt about its actual influence on his consciousness, which he refers to in the plural as comprising several layers that do not amount to a single cohesive being. The space created by the city in the mind of the author persists in its relentless, pestering demand to return there for reasons unclear to him that apparently stem from powers beyond his control. His return to the memory, or the return of the memory, *the return of the repressed*, like a strange dream, also plays out from within him, through the act of writing. The hold the city has on him is like a disease he keeps contracting. And as his recollection, the recurring overflow of his consciousness by the city, is experienced as a contagious virus, the author finds himself reverting time and again to the same persistent concern. The troubling concern to which he returns time and again is the issue of the sexuality of women. Her sexuality and passion, which drag down those who engage in the act of love, spell sickness or even death, whether of herself or of her man. The loss of the latter leaves her helpless in a patriarchal world. Such is the fate of the mother who loses her husband and thereby her entire world as is shown Nessim Hosnani's mother, Leila. Following the death of her husband, which could spell her liberation from an oppressive marriage, she is reduced to a mental and physical wreck.[115] Society won't have her any other way. It is not the woman's fault. The *mother-city*, the maternal being itself, is responsible for the wretched fate of its women. As Amaril, one of the minor characters in the *Quartet*, says in *Mountolive*. Alexandria is a city that leaves no other choice for women but to be abused.[116]

The figure of the mother wasting away at home following the death of her husband recurs throughout the work. It is the suffering mother, the mother whose agony justifies the journey of the prodigal son, the return of the hero, the return of the long lost son. The mother *is* the home, the city, the primeval Eden, the safe *Heimlich* without the uncanny connotations.

The return

Alas, even as he manages to return to this mother-city, he finds it is not the mother-city he left and remembered. In the *Quartet*'s last volume, *Clea*, Darley returns to Alexandria, the city he left at the end of the first volume. He is in fact summoned back to the city by Nessim Hosnani and finds himself embroiled again in the existential tangles created by his Alexandrian friends and in the labyrinthine being of the city itself. He returns to the city that he never left in his imagination and finds himself returning to an earlier version of himself. In his search for himself, he finds and then loses himself time and again within the mother-city of his consciousness. He asks himself how long he has been away, a question he finds impossible to answer. Time is no longer a loyal device to rely upon. The calendar proves futile as he looks at the pages and tries to recount his days. In fact, he realises that he had never truly left. He had been living in the Alexandria-of-the-heart. Having set out to chronicle the city and the actions of his friends, he finds he has failed. He cannot assume an observing position towards it. He is immersed in it, overwhelmed by its external and internal impact upon his mind.

Returning to the city means admitting the failure of his previous efforts to understand his experiences there. Balthazar's notes on the manuscript Darley wrote on Justine and Alexandria have proven him to be lacking and amiss in the second volume while the third volume offered the reader an "objective" glimpse into all that has taken place in the first two volumes. The narrator now returns to the city from a different point of view, which no longer presumes he can possess the truth. No longer does he know why or where he returns. He only manages to concede the intensity of the power that pulled him back, and his inferiority to it. This time around, he is aware that his journey to Alexandria is not without its past, or history. He refers to the presence of Cleopatra (c. 69–30 BC) and Hypatia (c. 350–417 AD), as well as to a more modern figure like French poet Arthur Rimbaud (1854–1891).[117] Delving into history does not ease his sense of disappointment; on the contrary, he feels like a ghost walking through his (partially false) memories and the memories of others. Returning to the city means returning to the memory of the city he has woven in his imagination. He returns to the city with the purpose of bidding it a final farewell.[118] But the city that welcomes him won't let him stay trapped in his dreams for long. It is a city in the grip of German artillery attacks during the Second World War. He arrives at the port while the city is under airstrike. The actual reality slaps him in the face and he must see it for what it is. Despite the harsh reality for a large portion of Alexandrians due to the war, Darley gradually returns to the personal experience where the city becomes an inner idiosyncratic cloister for him. Alexandria is no longer the shelled city, the city where his friends have lost property and status and sustained fatalities, but resumes its being as an inner arena for his existential struggles, which once again revolve around sexuality. The city, which for a brief moment went back to play an actual part in the world as a "real" city, rather than a mere poetic or liminal space, resumes its ritualistic proportions, as the narrator once again walks its streets. Walking around the city is wandering in writing in his city of his imagination.[119] The perverse sexual nature that he invests in the city and his relationship with it remains unchanged even after the years of apparent exile on the Greek island. The city is both a princess and a harlot. At once majestic and the anus of the world. It keeps throwing the same confounding and unsettling experiences at him, where the contrasts perhaps serve to ward off anything he is unwilling to bear. Thus, Durrell once again pronounces his conservative, separatist position. Alexandria is a city that serves him an arena to stage the sexual wishes and struggles of every British-born white writer who arrives in a city that embodies for him the *unheimliche*, exciting, intimidating sexuality and allows him to wade into unconscious parts of his psyche. It could be any other city. Alexandria as an actual being, rather than a mere receptacle for his consciousness, eludes the author's gaze.

Such a representation of Alexandria as the Other city allows Durrell to keep it at bay as a familiar maternal place that retains him as a child bonded to his mother by a childlike sexuality. The sexuality that the author finds (or invents) in Alexandria is a mature sexuality with perverse undertones that attest to his effort to get away from the familiar conservative patterns of his upbringing. Alexandria is like a mother in whom he can find the object of his love and hate at one and the same time, as well as the space he so wishes to get away from – the space represented in his consciousness by the *English death* of which he wrote in *The Black Book* (1938).[120] Alexandria is everything that any homeland (be it India, England or any other real country) neither was nor could be. It is the place where sexuality is allowed free rein, shaking free of the moral inhibitions that subject him to the religious patriarchal dictate and detaches it from any familiar moral order. This free rein is evident in the key reference that Durrell assigns to perverse sexuality in several places in the *Quartet*: his lengthy quotes from Marquis de Sade's novel, *Justine, or The Misfortunes of Virtue*, the epigraphs to two of the *Quartet*'s volumes, the actual choice of the name Justine for the key female protagonist, and in the diverse sexual contents he weaves into the tetralogy.

De Sade is insinuated into the pantheon of the narrative voices. His presence there lends the sexual regression its full intensity. The French psychoanalyst Janine Chasseguet-Smirgel (1928–2006) argues that everyone harbours *a perverse nucleus* that could manifest under certain circumstances.[121] She defines perversion itself as a challenge to all sexual and generational differentiations. As she demonstrates in her analysis of de Sade's aforementioned book, it is the undermining and obliteration of these two differentiations, gender and generation, that create the immense perversion experience that attends the entire book, where man allows all his repressed sexual desires free rein, with conscientious and social impunity. She conceptualises this experience as *the anal world*, which sees all sexual and generational differences transgressed while sexual intercourse can be exercised by any two people, irrespective of any previous kinship relations.[122] The single most representative experience of *the anal world* is the one encapsulated in the successful offensive against the mother and motherhood: "The creature I am destroying is my mother."[123] According to Chasseguet-Smirgel, this offensive, which sees man succeed in overcoming his mother and the creation of *the anal world*, opens up the door for creating a new world order to replace the Oedipal world where man tries to overcome his father, while his predestined failure dictates the social order that accepts the supremacy of the law. In the Oedipal world, which rests on relations of separation and differentiation, the kinship and incest laws establish these boundaries. In *the anal world*, all boundaries crumble to make way for a new order that endeavours to earn man's recognition of the experience where his sexual desires are neither subjected to repression or denial nor to the governing mechanisms that beget the incest laws; rather, they gain expression and recognition in the conscious reality. In this world, everything goes.

The Alexandria Quartet's author resorts to de Sade so as to pronounce an optional wish to destroy the world of his homeland, which holds his past and family. Lawrence

Durrell's Alexandria in the *Quartet*, the mother-city, is a liminal space where man experiences, even fleetingly, the prospect of a different world where his forbidden and repressed wishes come true. In a world as such he could have denied the pain he experiences due to separation, desertion or betrayal and thereby overcome his castrated position in the world. In such an alternative reality, Alexandria's liminal space transpires as a place where man does not enjoy the fruits of Oedipal sexuality that allows him evolve into a person wisened by the pain of breakup, desertion and loss.

In the Oedipal world that Darley ultimately inhabits, sexual experiences wound the individual. He is left alone with the legacy of the past, while the road stretching ahead won't allow him to form significant human relations. He survives, solitary yet alive and kicking and most importantly, writing. The final paragraph of the work, at the conclusion of the fourth volume, leaves no doubt about the future summoned by the author for the protagonist. Darley finds himself sitting down to his writing desk and beginning to write. He feels he is engaging in an ancient and sacred act which he is just the medium through which words will be written. Words which are laden with meaning, words of beginning. *Once upon a time*. Four words which symbolise for him the four faces of his friends, perhaps even the four volumes of the *Quartet* itself. He begins to write and feels the universe echo his tremendous effort. He is again on the eternal and precious quest for meaning.[124]

Writing is the author's last and only resort to realise his wish of returning to the *mother-city*, his lost homeland, the primeval experiences that chart his journey with magnetic forces that he cannot resist. He sits down to write the mythical first words, *once upon a time*, and feels the intensity of his consciousness succumbing to this trope. Whether he writes another novel, another version that follows the protagonist as he returns to his city, or whether he engages in letter-writing, as befitting the exiled writer he is shaping up to be, it is writing that will plot his course in his inner journey. Writing becomes his life and will entrap him again in the recesses of his consciousness. The boundaries between the fictional and biographical elements, between what *really* happened and that which has been written as *the truth*, will once again become the creative platform whereupon literature is written.

Notes

1 Steiner, George, 1961, *The Death of Tragedy*, London: Faber & Faber, p. 13.
2 Durrell, Lawrence, 1957a, *Justine*, London: Faber & Faber, p. 63.
3 Pedaya, Haviva, 2011, *Walking Through Trauma: Rituals of Movement in Jewish Myth, Mysticism, and History (Hebrew)*, Tel Aviv: Resling Publishing Ltd., p. 11.
4 Durrell, Lawrence, 1980b, *A Smile in the Mind's Eye*, London: Wildwood House, p. 26.
5 Nin, Anäis, 1967, *The Journals of Anäis Nin, Vol. Six 1955–1966*, London: Quartet Books, p. 129.
6 Alexandre-Garner, Corinne, 1997, "The Enigma of the Quartet", in Ilbert, Robert, ed., *Alexandria 1960–1980: The Brief Life of a Cosmopolitan Community*, Alexandria: Harpocrete Publishing, pp. 162–167.
7 Adam, Peter, 1987, "Alexandria Revisited", in *Twentieth Century Literature, 33/3*:395–410. In this article Peter Adam describes his 1977 Alexandria visit alongside Durrell,

ahead of a prospective filming an adaptation of one of his books. Durrell himself mixed, and allowed others to mix, his own biographical experiences in Alexandria and the experiences described in the *Quartet*.

8 Bachelard, Gaston, 1994, *The Poetics of Space*, trans. Maria Jolas, Boston: Beacon Press.

9 For further reading regarding the development of the concepts of the school of Object Relations that have developed the idea which originated with Freud's *Mourning and Melancholia*, read Jay Greenberg and Stephen Mitchell's book *Object Relations in Psychoanalytic Theory*, published by Harvard University Press in 1983.

10 Bollas, Christopher, 1991, *Forces of Destiny*, London: Free Association Books, 93–113.

11 In his original description, Bollas refers to the spatula as the actual object. In that, he echoes D. W. Winnicott's elaborate descriptions of his work as a paediatrician and psychoanalyst in Britain when the baby's use of the spatula was part of his diagnostic and therapeutic method. For further reading refer to Winnicott, D.W., 1971, *Therapeutic Consultations in Child Psychiatry*, London: Karnac Books.

12 In an essay written to mark *Justine*'s fiftieth anniversary, Egyptian journalist Mona Amis wrote that even though Durrell had been inspired by political events in Egypt and despite the just claims that viewed his perspective as representative of the imperialist outlook, it was important to remember that Durrell had intended nothing beyond the mythologisation of his personal experience, while any attempt to view him as an historian of his period missed the opportunity to enjoy the poetical and psychological merit of his work (Amis, 2007, pp. 1–5). An earlier critical view was expressed in Manzalaoui, Mahmoud, 1962, "Curate's Egg: An Alexandrian Opinion of Durrell's Quartet", *Etudes Anglaises*, 15:248–260. Other important essays supporting that criticism are: Halim, Hala, 2013, *Alexandrian Cosmopolitanism: An Archive*, New York: Fordham University Press and an essay she contributed in 2006 "The City as Feminine Principle: The Feminization of Alexandria in Durrell's Clea", *Deus Loci*, 10.

13 Howarth, Herbert, 1972, "Durrell Snapped in a Library", *London Magazine*, 12:71–84.

14 Morcos, Mona, 1967, "Autobiographical Elements in the *Alexandrian Quartet*", *Modern Fiction Studies*, 13:343–359.

15 Morris, Jan, 2012, "Introduction", in *the Alexandria Quartet*, London: Faber & Faber, pp. 4–9.

16 The term Durrell himself used to describe his attitude to those places is Spirit of Place. In a collection edited by Alan G. Thomas in 1969 by that title, one can find an extensive selection of letters and essays that Durrell wrote about the places he resided in. Durrell, Lawrence, 1969, *Spirit of Place: Letters and Essays on Travel*, ed. Alan G. Thomas, Mount Jackson: Axios Press.

17 Hashem, Evine, 1991, "The City: The Unifying Element in Durrell's Justine", in Gindi Hoda, ed., *Images of Egypt in Twentieth Century Literature*, Cairo: University of Cairo, pp. 77–89.

18 Bode, Carl, 1961, "Durrell's Way to Alexandria", *College English*, 22/8:531–538.

19 According to MacNiven, Durrell had indeed considered of placing the story in Athens but changed his mind as he was advised that this might upset his Greek friends. MacNiven, Ian S., 1998, *Lawrence Durrell: A Biography*, London: Faber & Faber, p. 322.

20 Ibid, p. 585.

21 MacNiven, Ian S., ed. 1988, *The Durrell-Miller Letters, 1935–1980*, London: Faber & Faber, p. 18. The use of capital letters is in the original.

22 Durrell, Lawrence, 1962, *The Alexandria Quartet*, London: Faber & Faber, p. 7.

23 This letter, early on in the rich correspondence between the two, can be read as Durrell's credo. In it, he expresses many ideas he will spend a lifetime developing and expressing. The relationship between young Durrell and the older Miller is one of the formative relationships in Durrell's life. Durrell first wrote to Miller after reading his *Tropic of Cancer*, a book he claimed changed his life. What began as a wide-eyed fan letter, soon developed to a mature and rich friendship, mostly through letters, which lasted till Miller's death in 1980. MacNiven, Ian S., ed. 1988, *The Durrell-Miller Letters*, 1935–1980, London: Faber & Faber, p. 18.

24 MacNiven, Ian S., ed. 1988, *The Durrell-Miller Letters*, 1935–1980, London: Faber & Faber, pp. 42–43.
25 Durrell, Lawrence, 1980b, *A Smile in the Mind's Eye*, London: Wildwood House, p. 86.
26 A very short 1942 text entitled "The Heraldic Universe" by Durrell was reprinted in Durrell, Lawrence, 2015, *From the Elephant's back: Collected Essays & Travel Writings,* Gifford, James ed., Edmonton: The University of Alberta Press, pp. 103–104.
27 French: so to speak.
28 Durrell, Lawrence, 1980b, *A Smile in the Mind's Eye*, London: Wildwood House, p. 49.
29 MacNiven, Ian S., ed. 1988, *The Durrell-Miller Letters, 1935–1980*, London: Faber & Faber, p. 17.
30 Ibid., p. 20.
31 Durrell, Lawrence, 1957a, *Justine*, London: Faber & Faber, p. 129.
32 Storr, Anthony, 1988, *Solitude,* New York: Ballantine Books, p. 74.
33 Durrell, Lawrence, 1960, *Clea*, London: Faber & Faber, p. 153.
34 Gifford, James, 2003, "Durrell's The Revolt of Aphrodite: Nietzschean Influence", *Mosaic* 36/2.
35 Jones, Ernest, 1953, *The Life and Work of Sigmund Freud,* Vol. 1, New York: Basic Books, p. 356.
36 Nietzsche, Friedrich, 1967b, *On the Genealogy of Morals*, trans. Walter Kaufmann, New York: Vintage Books, p. 15.
37 Nietzsche, Friedrich, 1967a, *Ecce Homo*, trans. Walter Kaufmann, New York: Vintage Books, p. 218.
38 Durrell, Lawrence, 1957a, *Justine*, London: Faber & Faber, p. 13
39 Nietzsche, Friedrich, 1967b, *On the Genealogy of Morals*, trans. Walter Kaufmann, New York: Vintage Books, p. 42.
40 Nietzsche, Friedrich, 1967a, *Ecce Homo*, trans. Walter Kaufmann, New York: Vintage Books, p. 233.
41 Durrell, Lawrence, 1957a, *Justine*, London: Faber & Faber, p. 13.
42 Nietzsche, Friedrich, 1967a, *Ecce Homo*, trans. Walter Kaufmann, New York: Vintage Books, p. 240.
43 Ibid., p. 261.
44 The term was coined by Melanie Klein and appears throughout her work. For further reading – Klein, Melanie, 1946, "Notes on Some Schizoid Mechanisms", in *The Collected Works of Melanie Klein,* Vol III. London: Hogarth Press and The Institute of Psycho-Analysis, pp, 176–200.
45 Zahaln, Anne, 1986, "The Destruction of the Imperial Self in Lawrence Durrell's The *Alexandria Quartet*", *Perspectives on Contemporary Literature*, 12:3–16.
46 Barthes, Roland, 1972, *Mythologies*, trans. Lavers Annette, New York: The Noonday Press, p. 96.
47 MacNiven, Ian S., 1998, *Lawrence Durrell: A Biography*, London: Faber & Faber, pp. 265–267.
48 Deep, Marquis, 1991, "Mahfouz and Durrell", in Gassick Trevor, ed., *In Critical Views on Naguib Mahfouz*, Washington, DC: Three Continents, pp. 27–37.
49 Durrell, Lawrence, 1957a, *Justine*, London: Faber & Faber, p. 153.
50 Festa-McCormick, Diana, 1979, "Durrell's *Alexandria Quartet*: A Whore Amongst Cities", in *The City as Catalyst: A Study of Ten Novels*, Cranbury, NJ: Associated Universities Presses, pp. 158–176.
51 Durrell, Lawrence, 1958a, *Balthazar*, London: Faber& Faber, p. 56.
52 Bhabha, Homi, 1992, "The World and the Home", *Social Text*, 31/32:141–152.
53 JanMohamed, Abdul R., 1985, "The Economy of Manichean Allegory: The Function of Racial Differences in Colonialist Literature", *Critical Inquiry*, 12:59–87.
54 Miller, Henry, 1945, *The Air-Conditioned Nightmare*, London: Granda Publishing.
55 MacNiven, Ian S., 1998, *Lawrence Durrell: A Biography*, London: Faber & Faber, pp. 232–305; Bowker, Gordon, 1997, *Through the Dark Labyrinth: A Biography of Lawrence Durrell*, London: St. Martin's Press, pp. 138–166.

56 Durrell, Lawrence, 1960, *Clea*, London: Faber & Faber, p. 24.
57 Adam, Peter, 1998, "Everything Comes Right", in Earl Ingersoll, ed., *Lawrence Durrell: Conversations*, Cranbury, NJ: Associated University Presses, pp. 163–170.
58 Williams, Gwyn, 1987, "Durrell in Egypt", *Twentieth Century Literature: A Scholarly and Critical Journal*, 33:298–302. See also a series of photographs portraying the coastal life of Alexandria and the city's hedonism. Moreno, Elie, 2011, "Once Upon in Egypt: Beaches and Bikinis from When Alexandria Was Club Med", *Foreign Policy*, April 27, pp. 36–48.
59 Jasanoff, Maya, 2005, "Cosmopolitan a Tale from Ottoman Alexandria", *Common Knowledge*, 11/3:393–403.
60 Haag, Michael, 2004, *Alexandria, City of Memory*, London: Yale University Press, pp. 87–143.
61 Porter, Roger, 2001, "Autobiography, Exile, Home: The Egyptian Memoirs of Gini Alhadef, Andre Aciman and Edward Said", *Biography*, 24:302–313.
62 MacNiven, Ian S., 1988, *The Durrell-Miller Letters 1935–1980*, New York: New Directions, p. 172.
63 MacNiven, Ian S., 1998, *Lawrence Durrell: A Biography*, London: Faber & Faber, p. 265; Bowker, Gordon, 1997, *Through the Dark Labyrinth: A Biography of Lawrence Durrell*, London: St. Martin's Press, p. 140. In addition, among other pursuits, Durrell was working at the time on *The Book of the Dead*, a novel that he had started writing before the war, its first manuscript left behind with his flight from Crete. The new version of this book had its focus on incest. Excerpts of this book, which had never been completed and which Durrell deemed unpublishable in Britain, found their way into the *Quartet*.
64 Even though the couple divorced in 1956, following nine years of marriage, Eve saw Durrell, even after his death, as the man who had helped her out of the subjugation of life with her conservative parents in Alexandria. She spent the greater part of her life in London and returned to Alexandria aged eighty. In an interview with Michael Haag she made a point of citing Durrell as the catalyst for her liberation process as an independent woman (Haag, Michael, 2009, "To Alexandria with Eve Durrell", in *Deus Loci*, 11: 3–6).
65 MacNiven, Ian S., 1988, *The Durrell-Miller Letters 1935–1980*, New York: New Directions, p. 170.
66 Durrell, Lawrence, 1969, *Spirit of Place*, Mount Jackson: Axios Press, pp. 99–100.
67 MacNiven, Ian S., 1988, *The Durrell-Miller Letters 1935–1980*, New York: New Directions, p. 159.
68 Ibid.
69 Ibid.
70 Ibid., pp. 160–161.
71 Durrell, Lawrence, 1969, *Spirit of Place*, Mount Jackson: Axios Press, pp. 101–102.
72 MacNiven, Ian S., 1988, *The Durrell-Miller Letters 1935–1980*, New York: New Directions, p. 164.
73 Ibid., pp. 167–170.
74 Ibid., p. 174.
75 Ibid., p. 180.
76 Bowker, Gordon, 1997, *Through the Dark Labyrinth: A Biography of Lawrence Durrell*, London: St. Martin's Press, p. 139.
77 Durrell, Lawrence, 1957a, *Justine*, London: Faber & Faber, p. 18.
78 Nietzsche, Friedrich, 1967, *Ecce Homo*, trans. Walter Kaufmann, New York: Vintage Books, p. 261.
79 Durrell, Lawrence, 1957a, *Justine*, London: Faber & Faber, p. 13.
80 Durrell, Lawrence, 1958a, *Balthazar*, London: Faber & Faber, p. 13.
81 Bachelard, Gaston, 1994, *The Poetics of Space*, trans. Maria Jolas, Boston: Beacon Press, p. 14.
82 Durrell, Lawrence, 1958a, *Balthazar*, London: Faber & Faber, p. 152.
83 Kristeva, Julia, 1991, *Strangers to Ourselves*, trans. L. S. Roudiez, New York: Columbia University Press, p. 26.
84 Durrell, Lawrence, 1957a, *Justine*, London: Faber & Faber, p. 13.

85 Callisto (Ursa Major) was the daughter of Lycaon, king of Arcadia. In her youth she pledged allegiance to goddess Artemis and took the vow of virginity. One day, while strolling around the woods, she was observed by Zeus, who lusted for her and raped her. The rape resulted in the birth of Arcas. Zeus knew that if his wife Hera was to find out about this liaison she would harm Callisto and her son, and therefore turned Callisto into a brown bear and took her away from her son. Bear Callisto kept wandering the woods looking for her son. One day she noticed him and, overcome by joy, forgot she no longer bore human semblance and walked up to him. Arcas drew out his sward in self-defence. Zeus observed the whole scene from high on the Olympus and was overcome with remorse. To avert the tragedy, he turned Callisto and Arcas into constellations. Hera nevertheless found out the truth and in order to punish the mother and son asked god Oceanus to forbid the two from bathing in his waters so they remain forever up in heaven. Arcturus (Guardian of the Bear) was created by Zeus to guard these two constellations against further feats of revenge by Hera.

86 Job 9:9, JPS 1917 Edition.

87 Job 38:32, JPS 1917 Edition.

88 Durrell, Lawrence, 1958a, *Balthazar*, London: Faber & Faber, p. 183.

89 Durrell, Lawrence, 1957a, *Justine*, London: Faber & Faber, p. 245.

90 Ibid., pp. 13–14.

91 Freud, Sigmund, 1954, *The Origins of Psychoanalysis: Letters to Wilhelm Fliess, Drafts and Notes 1887–1902*, Marie Bonaparte, Anna Freud and Ernst Kris, eds., New York: Basic Books, pp. 288–289.

92 Ibid.

93 The story behind Freud and Fliess's relationship is highly complex and has been the subject of several studies. The two men met on the recommendation of Josef Breuer (1842–1925), Freud's mentor and the co-author of the *Studies on Hysteria*. An initially passionate, warm relationship, it has been historically seen to involve latent, repressed homosexual elements. Both Freud and Fliess confessed at the time, as shown by the letter, that they perceived the individual to be a fundamentally bisexual creature. The rift between the two transpired after Freud realised that Fliess was refusing to relinquish some of his theories that upheld, among other things, the importance of the nose as a component of human sexuality, as well as the periodicity of masculine sexuality. The relationship was severed in 1904, while Freud refused to comment on it throughout his life and even ordered to destroy his letters to Fliess. The letters, which are now held at the library of the Hebrew University, Jerusalem, were purchased by Freud's pupil Marie Bonaparte from Freud's widow. Freud asked that she destroy them, but she managed to do otherwise and made sure to deposit them in a Switzerland bank vault. For further information regarding this period and others, reading either Ernst Jones' (1879–1958) loyal, three-volume biography, published between 1953 and 1957, or Peter Gay's more critical biography published in 1988, is a good start.

94 Durrell's *The Black Book*, faced the censorship's scourge for years and was even banned for publication in the US. Even later poems and of course the *Quartet* faced potential censorship while Faber & Faber's editor, T. S. Eliot himself, gently suggested that Durrell should omit some words so he did not have to do it himself (Armstrong, James, 1996, "Banned in America by the U.S. Customs Officials", in *Bibliographical Society of America*, 34: 230–256).

95 For further discussion of this, refer to Gifford, James, 2007, "H.D.'s Hirslanden Notebooks & Durrell's Claudia: Occult Modernism Across the Curtain & in the Mirror." In *ANQ: A Quarterly Journal of Short Articles, Notes, & Reviews* 30.3:145–149.

96 Turner, Victor, 1969, *The Ritual Process*, New Brunswick and London: Aldine Transaction.

97 Durrell, Lawrence, 1957a, *Justine*, London: Faber & Faber, p. 197.

98 Ibid., p. 24.

99 Ibid., p. 62.

100 Ibid., p. 68.

101 Durrell, Lawrence, 1960, *Clea*, London: Faber & Faber, p. 56.

102 Durrell, Lawrence, 1957a, *Justine*, London: Faber & Faber, p. 242.
103 Durrell was deeply impressed by Groddeck's thought and in 1979 even wrote the introduction to the English edition of Groddeck's 1977 book, *The Meaning of Illness: Selected Psychoanalytic Writings*.
104 MacNiven, Ian S., 1988, *The Durrell-Miller Letters 1935–1980*, New York: New Directions, pp. 169–170.
105 Groddeck, Georg, 1977, *The Meaning of Illness: Selected Psychoanalytic Writings Including His Correspondence with Sigmund Freud*, London: Hogarth Press and The Institute of Psycho-Analysis, p. 16.
106 Durrell, Lawrence, 1957a, *Justine*, London: Faber & Faber, p. 34.
107 Durrell, Lawrence, 1958a, *Balthazar*, London: Faber & Faber, p. 58.
108 Groddeck relied on this proposition when developing a method to treat physical illnesses and disabilities with a psychoanalytic technique. Although his legacy failed to strike roots in practice, he is considered to this day to be the father of the psychosomatic approach.
109 In his first letter to Freud, Groddeck expressed the fear (perhaps hope) that Freud will forbid him to practice psychoanalysis (as he had apparently received no appropriate training), and thereby also showed Freud to be a father figure for him. Not only did Freud not forbid him, he even encouraged him to pursue his work, introduced him into the International Society, arranged for his essays to be published in periodicals and even mentioned the term It coined by Groddeck, and Groddeck himself, in his 1923 essay entitled "The Ego and the Id."
110 Groddeck, Georg, 1977, *The Meaning of Illness: Selected Psychoanalytic Writings Including His Correspondence With Sigmund Freud*, London: Hogarth Press and The Institute of Psycho-Analysis, p. 11.
111 The original German term that both Freud and Groddeck used is *das ich*.
112 Groddeck, Georg, 1977, *The Meaning of Illness: Selected Psychoanalytic Writings Including His Correspondence with Sigmund Freud*, London: Hogarth Press and The Institute of Psycho-Analysis, p. 32.
113 Freud, Sigmund and Andreas-Salomé, Lou, 1966, *Letters,* Pfeiffer, Ernst, ed., trans. Robson-Scott, William and Elaine, New York: Harcourt Brace Jovanovich, Inc., pp. 63–66.
114 Groddeck took pains to stress that by that he was not referring to the concept of the unconscious, which he deemed a human development rather than a manifestation of it.
115 The circumstances surrounding the death of Leila's husband accurately resonate those surrounding the death of Durrell's own father.
116 Durrell, Lawrence, 1958a, *Balthazar*, London: Faber & Faber, p. 132.
117 Cleopatra was the last Macedonian queen to reign over Alexandria before it was overtaken by Roman Empire. Legend has it that she took her own life so as to avoid being captured by Roman Caesar Octavian. Hypatia was a Greek philosopher who lived in Alexandria during Roman rule. Her murder symbolised the struggle between the Greek enlightenment and Christian fanaticism. Arthur Rimbaud was a French poet whose tragic life inspired many writers. He gave up writing and wandering the world, Alexandria included.
118 Durrell, Lawrence, 1959, *Clea*, London: Faber & Faber, p. 12.
119 Ibid., p. 63.
120 More will be written of this book in the next chapter. It was the first one considered significant by Durrell, which earned him for the first time critical favour among writers like T. S. Eliot, follows the experiences of a young English writer struggling with the sexual oppression experience of 1930s England.
121 Chasseguet-Smirgel, Janine, 1984, *Creativity and Perversion*, London: Free Association Books, p. 3.
122 Ibid., p. 27.
123 De Sade, Marquis, 2008, *Justin or the Misfortunes of Virtue*, New York: Castle Books, p. 5.
124 Durrell, Lawrence, 1960, *Clea*, London: Faber & Faber, p. 282.

5

THE SECRET WOUND

The concluding chapter of my study will explore some aspects of Durrell's life that I find pertinent to a richer reading of the *Quartet*. In it, I search for what Julia Kristeva described as *The Secret Wound*, which challenges and haunts the wandering stranger.[1] It is by no means an attempt to explain his life through the *Quartet* or vice versa. Nor is this chapter a comprehensive or exhaustive biographical study. Any keen Durrell scholar will easily find that I have omitted many details of Durrell's life. I have taken the liberty of choosing certain details which I believe are significant when reading the *Quartet*. I believe that the details I have left out deliberately or unknowingly do not impoverish or alter the drawing I am trying to sketch of the *Quartet* in the context of Durrell's life.

Lawrence George Durrell (1912–1990) neither wrote an autobiography nor kept an orderly diary. The apparent reason is that Durrell viewed that kind of writing as a waste of precious time he could dedicate to poetry, prose and play writing. He told Anaïs Nin, who kept a record of her entire life in a series of diaries, that his aversion to diary writing stemmed from his fear that such a pursuit would devour him. Whatever he had to say or write about his life could be found in his prose and poetry, he argued, thereby demonstrating the interweaving of biographical and fictional elements found in literature.[2] Durrell thought that a writer must keep his personal experiences appropriately at bay if he were to be able to write. "You must make the leap outside of the womb, destroy your connections . . . disguise the personal, even when employing the diary form."[3] Durrell was inspired in this manner by one of the writers he most admired, D. H. Lawrence.[4] His close friend and spiritual mentor and inspiration throughout their fifty years of acquaintance, Henry Miller, on the other hand, wrote most if not all of his corpus as a series of revealing autobiographical writings that seem to do away with the biography-fiction distinction.[5] Miller's writing tempts the reader to perceive his personal confessions as reflective of the "truth" regarding his life, and therefore draw a screen over the fictional elements that Miller incorporated in them. Durrell was wary and ambivalent about the presumption of telling the "truth" about his own life. On the one hand, it was Miller's autobiographical novel *Tropic of Cancer* (1934)[6] that provided the momentum to write *The Black Book* (1938). On the other hand, he often criticised Miller for his self-disclosure, which he found to have slumped to its lowest point with the publication of *Sexus* (1949).[7] In that novel, Miller's unchecked exposure reached such extremes, complete with lurid details of his sexual escapades, that Durrell questioned its literary merit. He argued that Miller's writing might have held a therapeutic value for Miller himself, but offered no literary value for his readers.

For Durrell, prose writing was the appropriate framework for his desired biographical disclosure, allowing him control over the biographical details that were incorporated into it. In his many interviews following *The Alexandria Quartet*'s success, he was mostly happy to address questions about his life, yet tended to offer different versions. "To all the questions you did not ask, I can only answer in the affirmative."[8] He perceived the truth of his life as a deck of magic cards which he laid out for the audience to draw as they willed. He took an almost unlimited licence to render his life into fiction. He would joke about this penchant for inventing his life.

Durrell was of the view that concrete and honest disclosure of his life, such as Miller apparently exercised, would compromise the fountains of his art. In his book *A Smile in the Mind's Eye*, written in 1980, a decade before his death, Durrell expressed his fear of destroying the object of his writing with an actual reference to one event or another. "The minute you try to say something explicit about it you damage it, like clumsily trying to pick up a rare butterfly in your fingers."[9] Durrell feared that a style that was too forthright, intrusive and revealing would compromise his writing powers. This reflected his ambivalence towards Miller. On the one hand, he admired the latter's power to put right there on the table subjects that were considered taboo at the time, but, on the other, he could not write in a similar manner. In his quest for his authentic voice, a drawn-out process of many years, he found an intimate expressive form different from Miller's, a form that incorporated biographical and fictional elements. Whether it was a conscious choice he made as a writer or the outcome of his life circumstances and Anglo-Indian heritage that called for a more "cautious" kind of writing, Durrell opted to express his consciousness through his fiction prose rather than through autobiographical writing. An example can be seen in *Justine*, when he described Nessim kneeling by his bedside as an adult, mentally spellbound, an act he had not done since he was *twelve years old*, which is the age that saw Durrell himself spend his first year at the boarding school in England, a time later described by him as the great crisis of his life.[10] The scene is portrayed in the novel in a delicate manner, insinuating the mental anguish he experienced at that time. It is, as I will describe in the following pages, his *secret wound*, his deep sense of estrangement which began after he was sent away from his birthplace in India, sent away from his family, to England.[11]

In the late 1990s, two complete biographies were written by two separate scholars. The official biography, a thorough, considerate and finely detailed 801-page tome was authored by Durrell's friend, Ian S. MacNiven.[12] This biography takes an academic, appreciative account of his personal and literary relations. It is replete with many intimate details, such as Durrell's partiality to different kinds of wine or visits by friends and acquaintances to his home in the south of France. This biography takes a mostly sympathetic outlook, despite Durrell's notorious ways with women, and glosses over almost any criticism that has ever been levelled at the author. It is evidently the work of a man who shared close acquaintance with Durrell, edited some of his letters and writings for publication and loved him so much he was willing to turn a blind eye to some of his personal less savoury shortcomings.

The second biography was written during the very same years by Gordon Bowker, initially without knowledge of the other biography in the making.[13] The fact that this biography had been written almost simultaneously as its official counterpart meant that its author was denied access to Lawrence Durrell's archives, which affected the biography's writing and the nature of its focus. It was only as work was already underway that Bowker found out about MacNiven's official biography, but the publishers who had initiated the project encouraged him to complete it. This biography does not have the scope of MacNiven's and offers a more cursory account of Durrell's life. However, it raises several keen critical questions regarding Durrell's personal choices, his sadistic treatment of his women and his literary career.

A third important source of information concerning Durrell's life, though not strictly a biography, is Richard Pine's study, first published in 1994 and reissued in an expanded edition in 2005. It provides the most thorough survey and study of Durrell's oeuvre, as well as offering many valuable and critical biographical details.[14] No less valuable sources are the scholars Michael Haag and James Gifford who have been writing important and critical work about various aspects of Durrell's life and work.

Another source is the 1999 biography of his younger brother, Gerald Durrell, written by Douglas Botting.[15] Valuable information was also gleaned from the ample correspondences left by Durrell, including his more than fifty years correspondence with Henry Miller,[16] as well as his correspondence with writer Richard Aldington (1892–1962).[17] Additional sources are the memoir of Sappho Jane (1951–1985), Durrell's daughter by his second wife, published in 1985 after her suicide,[18] and writings by his close friends, Anaïs Nin and Henry Miller.[19] Further minor sources are two earlier studies of Durrell written by John Unterecker[20] and John Weigel at the height of Durrell's fame.[21] Last but not least are the numerous publications by Durrell scholars (known as *Durrellians*), many of whom belong to the International Lawrence Durrell Society. There are indeed too many to be given here the deserving credit.

The childhood *Kim* years

Durrell was born in northern India on 27th February 1912. His father Lawrence Samuel (1884–1928) and mother Louisa (1886–1964) were also born in India themselves, to parents of British descent. It was his grandfather, Samuel Lawrence Durrell, who was first posted in India in 1876 as part of his service with the British Army. On his mother's side, it was his great grandmother, the widow Louisa, who had moved to India in 1845 in the hope of finding a new partner. Her daughter of her first marriage, Louisa, married George Dixie and the couple begot Lawrence's mother.

Durrell was born to parents with an already complex sense of belonging. Though both Indian-born, the couple were part of a British community whose ties with the locals were colonialist by nature. They defined themselves as Anglo-Indian. Members of the Anglo-Indian community rarely married with the native Indians, for example, yet accommodated social and professional ties with them. The British Raj of India began with the seventeenth-century European imperialism, until India became a part of the British Empire. The complexities and significances of the multiple ties between England and India during that time are far reaching and beyond the scope of this study. It is a subject touched upon to an extent by Durrell's biographies. His family was indeed not directly engaged in the British military rule imposed upon India but rather part of the community of white individuals who lived in India and tried to earn a living. Nevertheless, they were part of the general colonialist culture that for centuries ruled India. Durrell himself engaged with his origins in a somewhat euphoric manner, while basing his identity as a child on Rudyard Kipling's (1865–1936) novel *Kim*[22]. Understandably, his memories of those early years in the different places where his family resided are naturally sensory, aesthetic and picturesque experiences, often citing no one but his close family. With the major exception of his *ayah*, his nurse-maid of whom he had very fond memories, the Indians as actual people seem to have been not greatly acknowledged in his writing other than as assorted exotic impressions. This impression of the locals surrounding Durrell is evident in *The Alexandria Quartet* as well, where the local Egyptian characters mostly form an indifferent aesthetic backdrop against which the plot is set. This perception of reality, with its implications for Durrell's development process as a descendant of a colonialist family, has a major role to play in how Durrell continued to perceive the places that he was later to inhabit as an adult, and shaped his attitudes to his surrounding population. He adopted an approach that seemed to draw on a Taoist-Buddhist notion that he referred to as *Quietism*, which allowed him to exercise existential alienation and was perhaps another example of the centrality of the *unheimliche* experience in his life.[23]

His birthplace was Jullundur (today known as Jalandhar), a small town in the northern part of the country. Durrell claimed to have remembered his moment of birth. The delivery was performed with forceps and once prised out of his mother's womb, he was left for long moments lying on a cold stainless steel table.[24] For him, this moment was his first experience of loneliness and alienation, and served as a portent. "I was even inconsistent in the womb my mother tells me, so there's no hope for change."[25] His mother told him that she had wanted an Indian doctor to be present at the birth, but his father had insisted that a woman of no previous relevant experience attend it. His second daughter, Sappho, wrote in her journals that Durrell had been born all sallow and for a brief moment had been taken for dead.[26] His mother told him that the birth itself had been protracted, causing him injuries. This memory drove Durrell in later years to delve into the works of Otto Rank, the Austrian psychoanalyst who was among Freud's pupils and colleagues.[27] Rank's treatment of the trauma of birth as a formative psychological experience in man's life served Durrell to form the notion that the violent nature of his birth affected his ability to feel at ease in this world. Durrell was described as a sickly baby who required devoted care to survive his first year. The memory of being sick, which he had eventually overcome, was to follow him later in life. The shadow of the sickness haunted Durrell, leaving its mark on his sense of self when he wrote *The Alexandria Quartet*, as I described in chapter four. The opening lines of *Justine* describe Darley as sick, wounded by his earlier experience. Later on, as he goes through the liminal space that Alexandria was for him, Darley finds sickness in the city, and in particular in the sexuality of its inhabitants which he attributes to the nature of the city as a *mother-city*. Several months after Lawrence was born, his father began work as part of the Buthidaung–Maungdaw railroad project in Rakhine, which became part of Burma upon India's declaration of independence. Thus began a period of wandering for the family in the sub-continent following his father's work. The town they moved to was situated near the Bay of Bengal, which meant an even greater isolation for the family. The area was cut off from other parts of the country and even the railroad connected two places along the bay, rather than connecting with the general railway network of India. And yet Durrell grew up enjoying relatively pleasant and comfortable physical conditions, within a sheltered environment that was nothing like the jungle *Kim*. Louisa Durrell kept local domestic help who tended to him all through the day and alleviated the burden of his care.[28]

In 1915, when Durrell was three years old, the Durrells once again relocated to a city north-east of Calcutta, in a region known for its hot climate. The family settled in the large city of Mymensingh, part of today's Bangladesh. It was a major cultural and social move, but the most significant change was the fact that Durrell's mother was pregnant again. His two biographers disagree on the reaction of three-year-old Durrell to the loss of his mother's undivided attention. MacNiven downplays the emotional intensity felt by Durrell following the birth of little Margery on November 1915 and notes that the exhilaration of the imminent Christmas helped Lawrence deal with his jealousy at his mother's focus on the baby. According to Bowker, Louisa Durrell was an anxious mother who avoided spending time away from her children and shunned social contact during those years so as not to lose precious time with them. He argues that the introduction of Margery into Durrell's life was not trivial for him, as it robbed him of her exclusive care.[29] Unfortunately, the baby girl did not live long and died at three months old from diphtheria, a prevalent respiratory disease at the time. Though infant mortality among that age group due to diseases was not uncommon in India, this death had harsh repercussions for the mental state of Durrell's mother.[30]

Louisa Durrell

There are several views upon the character of Louisa Durrell. An entry from the diary of Sappho, for example, noted the possessive nature of her grandmother and even likened the latter's relationship with Durrell to the one between a patient

(Durrell) and a nurse (his mother).[31] Sappho argues that, according to her father, his mother adored Florence Nightingale (1820–1910), and it was only after reading the biography of the renowned nurse that he had understood his mother's character and their relationship. Sappho describes this relationship as very close even when a long distance apart. This perspective is probably also informed by Sappho's relationship with her own mother, who she describes as a depressive woman indifferent to her needs. Durrell himself invests the mother figure with immense importance. Making no specific reference to his own mother, he writes to Miller in 1955: "it is mostly mother. She is the key – and she should devise the suitable disciplinary pattern for them (the children); without her they topple inside."[32]

Gerald Durrell, described their mother as a devoted, anxious mother who had dedicated her life to her children.[33] This account probably addresses one aspect of Louisa's personality. At the same time, according to Gerald, she also told him that prior to his birth she would drink gallons of champagne. Louisa's drinking dated back years before her pregnancy with Gerald, the youngest of her four children. Gerald, like Lawrence himself and their sister Margaret "Margo" Isabel Mabel Durrell (1920–2007), portrayed his mother as endlessly devoted to her family and their rock back in India, during their move from England to Corfu and even in her decision to make England her permanent home, where she remained a central axis in their lives.[34] Gerald pays her the following tribute in the opening of his famous book, *My Family and Other Animals*, where he described the four years, from 1935 to 1939, which the family spent in Corfu after Lawrence had talked his mother into leaving England:

> I should like to pay a special tribute to my mother, to whom this book is dedicated. Like a gentle, enthusiastic, and understanding Noah, she has steered her vessel full of strange progeny through the stormy seas of life with great skill, always faced with the possibility of mutiny, always surrounded by the dangerous shoals of overdraft and extravagance, never being sure that her navigation would be approved by the crew, but certain that she would be blamed for anything that went wrong.[35]

Botting, Durrell's biographer, described Louisa at length and tried to paint a comprehensive picture of her. Apart from being a devoted wife and concerned mother, he noted that she would sometime fail to behave as expected of a white woman of her class. Unlike many other women in her vicinity, she studied nursing and even practiced this profession and performed other menial works (including floor cleaning – which was very much below her status). Though perceived at times to be a frivolous and neurotic woman (traits that Lawrence Durrell would later put down to what he claimed were her Irish roots), Louisa also seemed to exhibit playfulness and willingness to face dangers, real or imagined. However, this portrayal is based on a rather unreliable evidence of an event where the family domestic help feared the presence of ghosts in the house, while Louisa, against their cautions, headed out into the dark woods on her own and "expelled" them.

On March 1917, about a year after baby Margery's death, Leslie Stewart (1918–1983) was born. He too, like Lawrence, was a sickly child, requiring the best of his mother's attentions. Louisa had to throw herself into caring for Leslie, at Lawrence's expense. Five-year-old Lawrence had to find himself other figures and activities in the house to spare himself the pain of solitude, which would nevertheless become his lifelong companion. In 1918, when he was six, the family moved to the town of Kurseong in the region of Bengal, where Samuel Lawrence was posted in his new capacity in the Darjeeling-Himalaya railway project. Despite its actual distance from the Indian border with Tibet or from any point within sight of the Tibetan mountains, Durrell had memories of looking over to the snowy Tibetan mountains from the town. "I was in a Tibetan dream until I was eleven years old . . . then began the madness of my life."[36] Such statements demonstrated Durrell's free use of biographical information, which he manipulated to suit the spirit of things he wished to convey. Later, Durrell would refer to that imagined vicinity to Tibet as a primeval homeland experience that had shaped his life. As Richard Pine wrote: "It was in the north-east, however, in Kurseong, that the young Lawrence Durrell began his lifelong attempt to locate his life of exile between the memories of his childhood and his colonial views of 'home'."[37] True or not was not really the point but rather his attempt to tell a good story. It was his subjective experience which shaped his sense of himself and inspired him to write the way he did, trying to find his way home.

Bowker wondered whether these frequent moves had actually been professionally motivated, as Lawrence Samuel's had enjoyed a lower salary in his new post. He assumed that the move was also spurred on by Lawrence Samuel's fear for his family given the emerging riots during those years against British rule.[38] A year later, when Durrell was seven, his sister Margaret was born. For him, this birth was another mark of the end of the age of innocence and his seamless coalescence with his parents.[39] When asked why it was the birth of his sister, rather than the earlier birth of his brother Leslie, that had marked for him the beginning of his solitude, Durrell failed to answer. Following the birth of Margaret, Lawrence was allowed even less time with his mother and was entrusted to his governess, whom he hated for her strict ways and habit of smacking him whenever he disobeyed her. His father was away at work while his mother had two infants on her hands, two-year-old Leslie and newly born Margaret.

Durrell stated that it was during those years that he had discovered reading. The solitude supposedly forced on him by his exclusion from his mother's lap made him rely on his inner world. The children's books that Durrell was exposed to during those years, like Rudyard Kipling's *Kim* and other adventure books like George Henty's (1832–1902) *The Lion of St. Mark*[40] or Rider Haggard's (1856–1925) books,[41] allowed Durrell to identify with characters of adventurous English boys. The protagonists in those books were scions of the authoritative imperialist British tradition, on the one hand, while demonstrating a burning desire for freedom and individualistic streaks.

Leaving for exile – the paternal imperative

In 1920, the family once again left their home and moved to Jamshedpur, at the heart of the plain surrounding Calcutta. If that was not enough to undermine what little stability Durrell enjoyed, a year later, aged nine, he was sent to the Jesuit boarding school of Saint Joseph's in Darjeeling, a long distance away from his family home. During his years at the boarding school, Durrell began to write. He would later cite his family's frequent moves as the root of his urge to travel the world, but until he was sent to boarding school, every change of location entailed the entire family moving together. For Durrell, moving to boarding school at nine was the first formative experience of banishment, which dogged him for years. Durrell wrote of the formative link between the experience of travelling and the reflective experience in *Bitter Lemons* (1957), the book written parallel to *Justine* when he thought that the experience of travelling has its rewards, not least because of the space it allowed the traveller for introspection.[42] This philosophical observation on the travelling experience allays some of the pain that must have attended that first separation from the family circle that cushioned Durrell until he turned nine, a circle he was severed from by his father's decision. Durrell stated that he had weathered the crisis with the help of his same-fated peers in the boarding school, but also thanks to his ability to withdraw into his rich inner world. MacNiven wrote that in a private conversation, Durrell had confessed that this move had been the first link in his lifelong solitude experience, which had nevertheless introduced him to writing, his passion, and provided him the space required for it.[43]

According to MacNiven, Durrell's parents were divided on the necessity of sending him to a boarding school. His father wanted Durrell to benefit from a better education, while his mother realised the emotional implications of separation for the boy, but did not have the strength to dissuade his father. Durrell was sent away as planned. His mother's failure to protect him from his father's wish to train young Durrell as the next generation in a patriarchal dynasty, which he viewed himself to be a member of, shaped Durrell's views of his parents in complex manners. His father remained a figure that cannot be defied, let alone ignore, while his mother was cast as the doting, devoted maternal mother who nevertheless could not prevail over the father's decision and was perhaps even complicit in sending him away. This position was seen by Durrell as an intrinsic maternal weakness and marked his mother, and other women, as the target of the displaced aggression he felt towards his father.

Two years later, at eleven, Durrell was sent by his parents from India to England, where he first attended a day school at Southwark and then a boarding school in Canterbury, as was the custom in the Durrell's social class.[44] England and the Anglo-Indian colony shared close ties and the affinity of the Anglo-Indian community whose families had immigrated in the nineteenth century was mostly underpinned by a fierce cultural and emotional bond with the Crown. Sending their eldest to be schooled in a traditional upper-class British setting seemed like the natural and right thing to do.[45] It secured the ongoing reign of tradition. The upper-class British education was seen as an inevitable rite of passage, even at the price of separation from the family. Moulting the childhood skin to make way for the new self to emerge from the rubble of memory is an inescapable fate. Thus dictated the British upper-class tradition to anyone who wished to become a gentleman.

As Durrell speaks through the voice of Mountolive, being educated was seen as a total departure from known reality. It was like entering a new and alien country where one would lose his bearings in the world. His previous identity and sense of self would be transformed and he would find himself assuming a new shape.[46] The timing too was carefully chosen. Durrell arrived at an age where his Indian environment started to infiltrate into his speech as well. According to his younger sister Margaret, it was the age when the soft, lilting Indian pronunciation of English started to insinuate itself into Durrell's speech, and his father wouldn't have it. It was of the uttermost importance that his son look and talk like a British gentleman rather than a little Indian.[47] There was no room left to consider the emotional implications of this separation on the young boy or for the entire family, at least not enough to affect the actual decision. While Louisa Durrell did at first raise her objection against him being sent to England, as she had done two years earlier, before his departure to Saint Joseph's boarding school, she again failed to change the paternal decision. Durrell was, by his own later admission, a "spoilt" child, that is, a child who struggled to part from his mother. The boarding school summarily severed that tie while forcing him to cope with loneliness and jealousy of his younger siblings, Margaret and Leslie, left cushioned in their mother's loving bosom. In one of his private conversations with MacNiven, while the biography was in the making, Durrell commented on his separation from his mother, in a rare revelation of pain: "I was terribly spoilt by my mother in India. Being exiled to England severed that bond."[48] In both cases, Durrell deemed the end result a betrayal and failure on his mother's part to protect him. According to Bowker, this experience offers an important insight into Durrell's sadistic treatment of his wives, lovers, Sappho and other women in his life.[49] He continued to act out the inner drama of his parents' betrayal with a sadistic, disparaging attitude to women in his life, while at the same time upholding an idealising façade of admiration to men, such as Miller, who served as father substitutes. As attested by his daughter Sappho:

> Father 'tells' me directly and not so directly that sex is about sadism . . . my childish question is why . . . my malevolent (frightened) father's answer is because women's sexuality is too frightening and disgusting not to be punished by men . . . Because he hates himself so much he's desperately trying to push this self-hatred on to me (women generally is the pattern).[50]

MacNiven and Bowker alike cite Durrell's being sent to England as the end of the freedom he enjoyed in childhood. The banishment to England was meant to symbolise his ancestral bond with the British homeland, but as Durrell would later write, the move achieved the opposite result and in fact imbued that *homeland* with dark and threatening connotations. From that time, *homeland* and *home* became *unheimliche* concepts for him, holding mainly ambivalence. In his last interview, conducted by Michael Dibdin at the behest of the *Independent* newspaper, Durrell said that, as far as his sense of belonging was concerned, he was doomed to a false life – neither Indian nor British, he had spent his entire life pretending about his identity and belonging.[51] This pretence failed to dissipate his wish to return to a place he could call his home, a wish that he expressed in the *Quartet* in many ways and through many characters. For example, his account in *Balthazar* of Nessim Hosnani's return to Alexandria following his studies in Europe betrays biographical elements from Durrell's own life: the waiting mother, the death of the father, and particularly the memories of the primeval experience that has faded into the recesses of one's consciousness.[52] Durrell was separated from his family by the paternal imperative. This imperative dictates that the son must accept his father authority and follow in his footstep: he must separate from his mother's love, from his family and geographical homeland, from his natural living environment, in order to undergo the initiation processes that will make a man out of him, a British subject, part of the social class of his father and his father before him. For that purpose, the father himself is willing to separate from his beloved son; the same son he hopes will represent him in the world and carry the torch of his ways and culture, in the name of some abstract, vague ideal of belonging.

This episode in Durrell's life is mythical in its structure and is reminiscent of the biblical Binding of Isaac. But the mythical expression does not end there: the immense importance invested by the author of *The Alexandria Quartet* in the influence of the environment on man, with its latent forces, draws in part upon the validity of the patriarchal imperative to *sacrifice* the son for a noble ideal. When the city of Alexandria inflates into mythical proportions thanks to her influence over her inhabitants, the residual life of boy Durrell peeps through the folds of its plot.

The death of the father

MacNiven is confident that Lawrence Samuel Durrell, Lawrence's father, wanted his son to attend a high-standard institution and enjoy the prospect of moving up the social ladder, even at the price of separation from his family, particularly given the importance the father invested in social status. He feared that staying in India, his son would remain part of the Anglo-Indian caste, considered inferior by the British Empire.[53] The Jesuit boarding school in India fell short of the father's requirements and therefore Lawrence embarked upon his schooling years in England in 1923. He himself identified with this wish on his father's part and his idealisation of his father was not compromised thereby. He stated that his father had only wanted the best for him and acted on superior motives of improving his son's standing. He even saw it as proof of his being the favourite son. As Durrell's father died before his younger siblings were old enough to carry the family tradition of attending boarding schools in England, Durrell was allowed to hold on to this sentimental view of his father. The father's figure remained impervious to criticism, at least consciously. But the figure of the father responsible for the separation appears in the third volume of the *Quartet*, when Mountolive describes how he left India when he was eleven years old, wondering if he will ever see his father again. The scene holds the very tension of the sense of betrayal of the son feeling rejected and abandoned by his father for reasons that seem incomprehensible to the young mind.[54]

Sappho wrote in her journals that, in conversations with her mother, Eve Cohen, Durrell confessed that his father had been a stranger. She notes how the process of gauging the effect of sending him to boarding school was etched in Durrell's memory. According to her, Durrell told her mother that when he was eight or nine, his father had asked him what he would want to do when he grew up. When replying that he wanted to write, Lawrence Samuel had looked at him proudly, saying that, if that was the case, he must receive better schooling than available in India. According to Sappho, this memory shows how Durrell managed to repress his pain at the father's decision to separate him from his family, by investing the father with noble intentions.[55]

The death of his father, five years after Durrell was sent away to England, was probably caused by the high mental stress involved in his position as adviser for the local railway company. This capacity, which he landed thanks to his previous achievements in railway engineering, meant Lawrence Samuel had to contend with local colleagues who were trying to outwit him. Several months prior to his death at forty-three, he probably contracted a brain tumour, though no official diagnosis was submitted. His health rapidly deteriorating, he became erratic. He was found drinking ink. He was devotedly nursed during those months until his death in 1928.[56] Durrell himself received the announcement in a telegram sent to his boarding school in England. In fact, since leaving India in 1923 Durrell had seen his father only twice, during the latter's visits to England. He himself would never return to India, though he had contemplated doing so. Durrell rarely wrote or talked of his father directly. This avoidance, which was unlike his manner towards other subjects, may suggest an inner distress that Durrell harboured in relation to him. His emotional avoidance of confrontation with him is like Isaac's difficulty of looking his father in the eyes as he sets out to sacrifice him, in this case, for the cultural imperative of maintaining and upgrading his social status, as embodied in the act of his banishment to England.

Bowker suggests that Durrell was careful in his attitude towards father as he perceived him to be weak and rather than risk expressing his ambivalence directly, he adopted different father figures. According to Bowker, Durrell's father had ranked low on the social status scale of his community. He had been referred to as a *failed babu* – *babu* being the Hindi and Bengali word of respect for *sir*.[57] Balthazar refers to the phenomenon when he describes the increasing population of local middle class Anglo-Indians who sought better education for their sons and sent them away to elite British universities. Balthazar derided that trend, saying that all that these returning sons brought back with them was a lowering of the standards, a trend he could see taking place all over the world.[58] Durrell might have hoped for a more educated father, yet realised that the latter's main power lay in his total identification with the British Empire and its penchant for geographic and economic expansion and political domination. One of his significant memories of his father, which he recalled in a 1976 *Radio Times* interview, harks back to a dinner where his father banged on the table with fervour and called: "My God! We must drive ahead! We must drive ahead and *win!*"[59] His passing away deprived Lawrence Samuel of the opportunity to see his aspirations for his son come true, while the untimely death left Lawrence without an anchor in the world. The paternal imperative *we must drive ahead!* which for Durrell symbolised the might of his father, was the same gesture that drew him away from the homeland experience he had enjoyed in India. This gesture was to reverberate throughout his life. Yet, it may also be that his father's untimely death relieved Durrell of a burden. Had his father stayed alive, Durrell could end up even more preoccupied with his wish of pleasing him and becoming the writer and gentleman he had wanted him to be, or he could learn that his father's wish was not about the realisation of his literary talent.

The English death and *The Black Book*

Durrell had spent five years on his own in England before the death of his father and his mother's subsequent final departure from India in 1928 to England with his younger siblings. Durrell spent a mere twelve years in England, from eleven to twenty-three, when he moved to Corfu with his wife Nancy. During his years in England he attended a private boarding school, where he was a fairly mediocre student. It was then that he discovered his passion for writing as a form to express himself.[60] He discovered the world of adult love and sex. He also discovered his sense of alienation. As he would write through the lips of Mountolive, it was in England that he was taught not to feel.[61] In that place where his father sent him, under the pretext of forging his affinity to his ancestral homeland, Durrell endured alienation. He could have embraced England and its time-old tradition, but it only evoked his intense objection. He had no wish to belong to this place that was forced upon him. For him, this belonging on his part marked his exile. His stay in England made him want to leave it. His ancestral place of belonging became a place to act out rituals of differentiation in his personal liminal process. England is the place that would define his exile as of that moment, as he wrote forty years later: "I am, and I remain, an expatriate. That vague sense of exile has never quite left me."[62]

The expressions of this exilic experience in relation to England can be found in what he deemed his first major successful novel, *The Black Book*. Due to its explicit sexual content, Faber & Faber refused to publish it at first.[63] It was first published in France, earning him the recognition of writers he admired, like T. S. Eliot (Faber & Faber's editor at the time) and Henry Miller. He spent almost a year and a half working on the book, from September 1935 to December 1936, shortly after he travelled to Corfu. The plot of the book takes place in London's Hotel Regina, and follows the experiences of its guests. The plot is delivered from two narrative perspectives, and in so doing predicts *The Alexandria Quartet*, which was to be written about twenty years later. The first narrative is that of Lawrence Lucifer, a school principal. The second narrative is that of Death Gregory, whose diaries Lucifer discovers at the Hotel Regina. The novel's setting against a hotel backdrop allows strangeness to exist undisturbed, and even serve as the main essence of the entire plot. Although the hotel's guests are mostly permanent residents, or at least long-term sojourners, the author refers to them as transient, passing events in the realm of the hotel. It is designed for people in transition, holiday or with no permanent abode. The type of habitation is ancient, cited as early as the Old Testament (Isaiah 10:29: "they are gone over the pass; they have taken up their lodging at Geba; Ramah trembleth; Gibeath-shaul is fled"). Its very existence attests to the wandering, nomadic aspect of mankind throughout history. The hotel, a place to pass away the night, is a temporary lodging that can also become a permanent home. The hotel offers refuge for people away from their permanent abode and caters for their basic needs. In this sense, the transient home as both a safe haven and a hiding place is another expression of the *unheimliche*, homely and yet strange. The hotel is the lodging of the foreigner, the refugee and the exile.

The novel opens with a reference to the beginning of the struggle, the Greek *agon*.[64] The very first few words, spoken by the narrative voice of Lawrence Lucifer, point out Durrell's intention: It is the destiny of man to fight and seek his existence. It is wintertime and the winter is lyrically, complexly illustrated, replete with rich language and metaphors. The winds of the island blow from the east, the Levant. We see the author charting the atmosphere of moving to and fro. The wind signals the course of movement, of the unhomeliness that descends on the homely place, harbouring a threatening presence. Beyond the scents it carries over from faraway places, the wind also upsets the place it pervades. The author describes it as an actual presence, churning the earth, hauling up clay from the depth of the ocean and scattering it in the air, thus interfering with the fishermen but also protecting the sea creatures. The wind keeps the secret. Set against the wind are sounds of classical music by Bach. The wildness of nature intermingles with the mournful atmosphere inspired by the music in Lawrence and his partner as they lie in bed, mourning the death engulfing them.

The emerging theme is death – the death of the Mediterranean Sea with its galore of colours, scents, sensuality, undertones and flavours. The Mediterranean summer is devoured by the ancient Greek wind that churns up from the depth of the sea and makes way for winter.[65] This is no incidental winter. It is a Greek winter, inspired by Shakespeare; *the winter of our discontent*. The reference is to *Richard III*, one of Shakespeare's early plays. The brother of the King, who is envious of the latter's reign, works relentlessly, forcefully and cunningly to seize the throne, even if it involves killing his brother and other relatives. Richard III is an invalid, a hunchback, feeling tormented by destiny. He is portrayed as an anti-hero representing the mythical struggle waged between free choice and fate. Durrell's choice of this reference from the play, before the great crimes of Richard III are committed, hints at the theme that preoccupies him, the theme of man facing an overpowering fate and the urge to overcome it, even at the cost of committing a crime or deviation. Man is a stranger in this world, his power to make a difference minimal. It is an experience of helplessness, of emasculation and eventually death, in the face of nature's tremendous display of life. It is on such a day that the author of the novel chooses to begin his work. A day of death, when he will be writing an *agon* for the dead, telling the story of the living.

The book follows two parallel plots of life and death: life is ironically represented by the character named Lawrence Lucifer, while death is represented by Death Gregory. Durrell later refers to this death experience as *the English death*. Lawrence Lucifer is on an island, his exile away from his homeland of England, where staying felt tantamount to death for him. It is only from this exile that he can process his memories through writing. Lucifer cannot understand why it is only on the island that he is able to do so. He does not know what makes the characters that inhabit Hotel Regina inspire his imagination in that stormy night to write his first real book.

The winter experience of the Greek island dredges up memories of winters in England, inhabited by the characters at the Hotel Regina. These are eccentrics, living on the verge of self-disintegration. It is a perverse connection to life that keeps them alive, a connection almost invariably underpinned by intense explicit sexual experiences.[66] It is a connection to life made on the verge of death, *the English death*. *The English death* is the Anglican British puritanism where Durrell's father sent his son at eleven and from which Durrell fled when leaving England. This metaphor is the key theme he must face when describing the experiences of the characters in his book, who reconstruct his own experience. The death about which he writes is worse than actual death. The spiritual death, the sense of *unheimliche* felt within the homely, feels graver for him than actual death. The experience of the homely is a deadening experience for him. The familiar constitutes a cramped world that offers no outlet, even in one's imagination. The author proclaims that the only way to escape death is through a sense of illumination, a light, but this is not just any light, but the light that heralds Christmas, the birth of Jesus. It is not necessarily a happy recourse, but it forms a transition from the sense of death that engulfs the narrator. The loathing for Christmas, for the feigned, phony merriment, is the way out.[67]

It is the loathing and aggression that allow the protagonist to break free from the death experience. Loathing allows the author to get away from the place he has experienced as deadening and describe it in a way that would not have been possible unless he had escaped. The loathing-driven experience of getting away turns the bond with the forced, loathsome homeland into a creative bond.

The sense of revelation found in exile links to the enlightenment in Christmas and symbolises the ambivalent relationship the author has towards his *unheimliche* cultural homeland. The hotel's residents are almost invariably socially eccentric characters. With the exception of two foreign students, all characters are unemployed or unfit for any work. They live hand-to-mouth, self-debasing and engaging in abject relationships with each other. They express their aversion to the values of society, which they inhabit as strangers anyway, as living-dead spat out by their environment and isolated in that transient-permanent lodge where they live as protracted sojourners.

In the portrayal of the hotel residents, Durrell begins to explore the theme of wounded sexuality he will later expand upon in the *Quartet*. The character of Lobo, for instance, a Spanish architectural student and a lodger at the hotel, is obsessed with sex as a way of defying the puritan, depriving homeland he has left. The exile from a permanent abode in the British homeland and the act of settling down in the temporary lodging allow the characters a compulsive engagement with sex. This sexual focus, another theme which will recur in the *Quartet*, immediately becomes aggressive towards women, who are portrayed as adversaries. The other characters are just as grotesque. Old Tarquin, for example, fosters an obsession for another character, Clare, a gigolo and dancer refusing to become the object of his adoration. The only characters to enjoy an empathic portrayal are the red-haired whore, Morgan the janitor and Miss Smith, Lucifer's black student, who studies, somewhat pertinently, the works of Chaucer.

In *The Black Book* Durrell explored his ambivalence, aversion and yearning towards his sense of home. This ambivalence continued to preoccupy him. Twenty years after completing *The Black Book*, and by then very far away from England, Durrell returned to those very experiences, the experiences of pain that wouldn't relinquish their hold on his mind, with *The Alexandria Quartet*. But now, at a distance, he was able to address them from a different perspective. He understands that he is a refugee from the prolonged painful experience that living in England had been for him. It is only because he loves life so much that he was able to survive it and seek a new home for himself.

Greece and the coming of age of the author

It is hard to tell when a writer finds his authentic voice. Durrell began writing as soon as he was able to literally do so. He wrote and published two novels (one under a pseudonym) and some slim volumes of poetry before he wrote *The Black Book*. I suggest though that it was in his Corfu years that his writing reached a certain maturity. It was in Corfu that Durrell found his authentic voice. Durrell wrote *The Black Book* in Corfu during 1935–1936, which was in fact the tale of his twelve-year exile in England (1923–1935), while work on *The Alexandria Quartet*, the tale of his Egyptian exile in 1941–1945, commenced in 1953 in Cyprus and completed in 1959, when he was already living in the south of France. The strong voice of a man who has finally managed to shake off the distress that dogged him over the years emanates from the letters of that period in Corfu. In this island he found his artistic home. The low-cost life in Corfu, coupled with the Mediterranean air, was an experience likened to life in heaven for Durrell.

> Today we rose to a gorgeous sunlight and breakfasted in it. . . . [S]ometimes I almost suspect the whole thing; I don't think I can yet really believe in it. . . .

> I'd like to tell you how many million smells and sounds and colours this place is, but my stock of superlatives would give out. . . . I'm so despondent to write a BOOK. Something with contours and blood and stuff in it. . . . I HAVE BEGUN TO BE A REAL WRITER.[68]

The experience of writing did not come easy even in this paradise. Having apparently figured out the course he wanted to pursue following Miller's immense influence, Durrell found that the tangible, emotional and sensual writing he strove to achieve wouldn't just come out flowing. The same emotional inhibitions that he had blamed on the British culture kept exerting their influence from afar. He likened the craft of writing to fine cotton-sewing, crochet.

> I've been very down in the jaw lately over this fucking book [*The Black Book*] which won't go as it should . . . it is like fine crochet, done at one dead level of emotion. . . . I find that half our trouble is bad emotion. This comes from shallow sexual experience I feel sure. . . . What I am for from now on is the essential male and female friendship uncomplicated by mirages and falsities and wish fulfilments.[69]

Crochet was very commonplace among women of the Durrells' social class. The appearance of this feminine term among a torrent of prickly, and even crude, masculine words points to Durrell's complex, contradictory experience during those years. Not one of his letters from the period shows any sincere, earnest acknowledgement of the part played by women in his life – his wife Nancy, his mother and his sister – in the fact that he has struck a creative, stable, supportive environment for his forays into "real" writing. Having completed his first novel, Durrell realised it was not how he wanted to write. The introduction to Miller's books made it clear to him that he must undergo transformation. This change came at an immense emotional and intellectual cost, which Durrell described as a rebirth experience, but had yet to acknowledge the contribution of the women in his life to the atmosphere that allowed him to apply himself to writing. Nevertheless, as will be detailed later, it was the efforts of women in his life that provided the suitable habitat, the appropriate nesting experience, which allowed Durrell to realise his life project, *The Alexandria Quartet.*

It was not just to the women in his life that Durrell was indebted for his literary rebirth. This birth also had a spiritual father – Henry Miller.

> When I first read *Tropic* I was delighted with it, not as a new bible, but because it bore out a few theories about writing that I had been trying to formulate. . . . *Tropic of Cancer* is the purest book written in our time . . . and also the most religious book.[70]

The biblical image employed by Durrell to illustrate the influence Miller had on him emphasises the intensity of the transformation he felt he must undergo so as to be true to the new father figure who permeated his world. Miller commanded an expectation and demand that call to mind those imposed by Lawrence Samuel Durrell when excusing sending his son away to boarding school in England as the only way to pursue his wish to become a "real" writer. In both cases, it was a call by a paternal authority that Durrell tried to comply with, so as to realise a vision that was to become his own. The toll exacted by this compliance and following is a sense of alienation with the emotional world that Durrell identified with his mother, as exemplified in the crochet image. Durrell rejected the suggestion that Miller's writing served as his gospel to follow, but with this rejection he conferred upon Miller the position of a mythological father figure whom one must either obey or rebel against. In his own description, Durrell was on the cusp of carving a whole new literary space.

> There is no one else on the horizon in England who seems to be developing into the same kind of faun. . . . So, when I Durrealize, please understand . . . I do not compete. By degree I may be lesser; by genus I belong to another race. . . . I am my own kind.[71]

In his book *The Anxiety of Influence*, Harold Bloom refers to the issue of originality in poetry and notes that every new poem is composed relative to previous poems: "the meaning of a poem can only be a poem, but another poem – a poem not itself."[72] Bloom claims that every poet ends up trying to find his original voice, but can only "appropriate" the poetry that has influenced him – while trying to overlook the intensity of this influence – to "expropriate" the work's origin. Bloom describes this pretence for originality as an inevitable process. According to Bloom, every work is a patchwork of other, previous works that come together, consciously or otherwise, in a different order so as to try to renounce their original stock. He says that the writer can never get away from his literary home and really leave it. In every original text, therefore, the texts that comprise it can be read, which Bloom refers to as *intertexts*. Durrell saw himself as one of a kind when he wrote *The Black Book*.[73] At the same time, it is possible to see from his letters from the period, the impact of Miller's writing was hefty. Miller's works empowered Durrell to examine his view of his own life, in this case, his life in England, and focus upon motifs that so enchanted him in Miller's 1934 novel *Tropic of Cancer*. Durrell found similarities between Miller's exile and his own. For both men, the ability to write how and what they wanted to was the product of being away from their homelands and resulted from their coping with the death experience that was threatening to consume them. As Durrell wrote to Miller in September 1936: "All the questions posed in literature since Marlowe mean the same thing. In my opinion *Tropic* is the answer to them . . . somehow you have to be a real exile to do things on that scale."[74] In the opening lines of *Tropic of Cancer*, Miller wrote of his days at the Villa Seurat (where they would both live when they shared a residence in Paris). He described the house as immaculate and obsessively ordered, and therefore totally dead.[75] These words are chimed by Durrell himself in *The Black Book* where he writes that he chose to begin his book on the day when he found that they were all dead.[76]

What is this death that Miller wrote about and Durrell tried to appropriate so as to describe his own experiences? In *Tropic of Cancer*, Miller explains that death is the undoing of all the fetters imposed by modern society on the free artist in an attempt to rob him of his authentic work. Miller wrote the book in Paris, where he had moved from the US at the age of forty, in his desperate quest for a non-oppressive life style. For him, being poor and often hungry in Paris was a liberating experience through which he found his literary and personal voice, following years of failed attempts. Durrell, who, as noted earlier, came upon Miller's book after leaving England, his "spiritual prison," could not have found himself a more suitable influence. He too experienced England as a spiritually deadening place. Thus *Tropic of Cancer* paved his way to write *The Black Book*. But Durrell also writes of another death than Miller's. When he writes about death, he also writes about his father's death. Two points briefly emerge: one is the emotional death of his father, encapsulated by his actual willingness to send the eleven year old Durrell into the exile and solitude of the boarding school. The second is his actual death, thus preventing Durrell from imbuing their relationship with the emotional experience that he expresses in his writing. It is doubtful whether Durrell could have expressed the full complexity of his emotional experience to his father had he been alive still, but the father's physical absence left him no choice but to express it through writing. When he is writing about *the English death*, he may well have been writing about *the death of the British* gentleman that his father wished him to be.

The time Durrell spent in the Mediterranean granted him the inner freedom he sought. He found his literary voice during those years and even felt "at home" again on the Greek island, but the Second World War interrupted this idyllic experience. Durrell lived in Corfu until 1939. One of the many highlights for Durrell during his time in Greece was Miller's visit, which Durrell wrote of enthusiastically.

> I have been more or less tongue tied: the war is like a great severance, and your voices sound muffled across the gulf. I have written to no one, because there is not an atom of comfort to be given. It is a huge symbolic contortion in which individual lives seem to lose their significance and shape. I am cut to the heart and womb.[77]

Together with Nancy, the two went sightseeing around Greece, but even this visit failed to lift Durrell's spirits in the face of the impending war as he wrote in a later letter to Miller: "At the moment everything is upside down and what with air raids and one thing and another I have hardly time to think. We are submerged in the struggle."[78] As the war broke out, his mother and siblings returned to England, while Durrell and Nancy moved to Athens in the hope of finding work there, as he did eventually when he was appointed to run a school in Kalamata. In 1940 their daughter Penelope was born and when she was just three months old the couple had to leave and escape to the Egyptian shores and the port city of Alexandria.

The abrupt, forced departure to Egypt interrupted a positive period of creativity for Durrell. During his time in Greece he experienced first-hand the Hellenistic culture he had hitherto only read of in the Romantic and Elizabethan literature. His writing started to embody his deepest intentions. He met Miller, whose personal and literary influence would attend him throughout his life. He enjoyed a high standard of living and a happy relationship with Nancy, and their daughter Penelope was born a few months before their forced departure. He therefore found in Greece the home he had been forced to abandon at eleven upon leaving India. When the war was over and Durrell left Alexandria, he set out on a series of posts as an employee with the British Foreign Office and British Council in the Dodecanese islands, Argentina, Yugoslavia, and Cyprus. It was only in 1958, following the meteoric success of the *Quartet*'s first volume, that Durrell settled in the south of France, which became his permanent home until his death in 1990.

The years of writing *The Alexandria Quartet*

Durrell wrote most of *The Alexandria Quartet* while already living in the south of France with, Claude, an Egyptian Jewess and descendant of the Menasce family, renowned in Egypt of that period thanks to its banking enterprises. Claude, a budding author, was born in France. Durrell met her in Cyprus in 1955, when she was still married to Tim Forde, an Irish businessman who travelled the world as part of his enterprises. Their two children, Barry and Diana, stayed with their father and accompanied him on his travels. Looking for a job at Durrell's office,[79] she was appointed at once to run the French division of the Cypriot radio services, thanks to her command of several languages. Their relationship soon flourished, not least when Durrell realised she knew some of his acquaintances in Egypt and came to appreciate her intellectual and literary merits.[80] He wrote to Nin that

> I have abducted a young woman, French, from Alexandria, who writes light novels in English, is very pretty, cooks and makes love like the Arabian Nights. Claude by name. . . . It was heartening for the first time in my life to find a woman who was almost more anxious for me to write than I was myself – and who was determined to get a job to keep me if I couldn't keep myself.[81]

The intense love between the two was underpinned by the centrality of writing in their lives. When meeting Durrell, Claude was busy writing her first novel.[82] Durrell himself, who had been busy for some years writing *Justine*, and failing to elaborate the book to his satisfaction, found in Claude an exquisite writing partner. She encouraged him to concentrate on his writing and the two would sit at their office facing each other, each with their own typewriter. Durrell pinned a large map of Alexandria on the wall and tapping into Claude's deep acquaintance with the city, charted the plot of the novel. MacNiven and Bowker describe Durrell's relationship with Claude as the most successful of Durrell's four marriages. He met Claude several years after separating from his second wife, Eve Cohen, who had suffered a series of severe mental breakdowns and frequent psychiatric admissions. The couple's daughter Sappho first lived with Durrell's mother, and once her father's relationship with Claude gained momentum, she moved in with them. She found in Claude a loving stepmother, who managed to deal successfully both with her fierce love for Durrell, her writing and the care of the shared household.

The love shared by the couple was neither perfect nor harmonious. Friends and acquaintances often reported that Durrell had not refrained from his flirtatiousness with other women, nor had he reined in his hot temper with his beloved wife, and that their relationship had been through some rocky patches. When Anaïs Nin visited their southern France home in 1960, she was left with mixed impressions. She described the household run by Claude as a warm, abounding place that mainly relied on her positive energies. Durrell himself struck her as self-absorbed, and she was disappointed to be left out of his circle of affection as he dedicated himself to writing and to Claude. She saw him as a man who had found his home. According to Nin, Durrell was no longer the same lost young man she had first met upon his arrival to Paris in 1937 to meet his idol, Henry Miller. She thought him to be a vacuous man with a shallow personality, whose writing promised more than it could deliver.

> Decided Durrell does not have a deep knowledge of character. It shows in this Balthazar, soi-disant psychiatrist. He promised relativity of truth but that lies in acceptance of subjectivity, and that means introspection, going inwards, which he has not done. . . . He lives in fiction. Like Henry, he invents. He does not see.[83]

The ten years that the couple spent together until Claude's sudden death from cancer in 1967 were the most creative and prolific of Durrell's life. With Claude by his side, he found his lost, primeval motherland. His relationship with her provided him the right blend of fierce love, with its inter-dependency elements, and the creative freedom to sound his literary voice. Their years together were his "homecoming" back to the intensive relationship with a loving, dedicated woman, perhaps not unlike his relationship with his mother until his first banishment from the family at the age of nine. His years with Claude allowed him once again to find "himself" in a beneficent, unfettered belonging experience, like the one he had enjoyed back in his childhood years in India. Seemingly in jest, Durrell noted during those years that Claude had written everything for him, even his love letters.[84] It is safe to say that it was Claude who managed to inspire Durrell to complete *Justine* and the *Quartet*. In all likelihood, had it not been for her support and guidance, no sequel (or sibling) would have been written for *Justine*. According to Michael Haag, it was Claude who told Durrell of the operations of arms trafficking to Palestine that her family on her mother's side (the Alexandria Menasce family) had been involved in during those very years that Durrell had spent in Alexandria.[85] It was the inspiration that Durrell needed to breathe life into his project of writing his multi-layered novel. Durrell, who wanted to protect the family's reputation and spare it the Egyptian regime's wrath (these were the *Lavon Affair*[86] days), used the facts provided to him by Claude but converted the identity of the masterminds behind the scheme to Coptic Egyptians.

Claude was all his dreams come true. In his letters to Miller he described her deep devotion and how she would type every single one of the books he had written during that period, including proofreading for all editions translated into French, German and Italian, which she was versed in. At the same time, she ran the household and saw to all his needs. During that very same period, she wrote three novels published by Faber & Faber in London. Apart from being the muse who allowed him to realise his literary life passion, she also served as the ideal mother. She is the key – and she should devise the suitable disciplinary pattern for them; without her, they topple inside. . . . Claude has the knack of joining forces with them and leading them from the inside, so to speak."[87]

Durrell mentions Claude's children three times in his correspondence with Miller, and even then it is only casually, in passing, while surrendering no further information other than the fact that the children spent their summer holidays with Durrell's daughters.[88] Durrell went into further detail about being torn between wanting to apply himself to writing and the burdensome duty of seeing to the children's needs. This grievance, needless to say, fell on the sympathetic ear of Miller, who struggled with similar hurdles. The two confided in each other about the burden of child-raising, coupled with their accelerated fame and the growing influx of visitors and letters, which combined to disrupt their focus on their writing.

The happy decade and the lost children

The ten years he spent with Claude seemed like the happiest in Durrell's life. He liked the south of France for its Mediterranean atmosphere, which he had pined for since he had left Greece. His work was published and earned the critical esteem and commercial success he had craved. But these years were tragically interrupted in 1967 with the death of Claude, several months after she had been diagnosed with advanced-stage cancer. Durrell never recovered from the blow in his remaining twenty-three years. The books he wrote during those years met with cold reception. Durrell did marry his fourth wife, Ghislaine de Boysson (1927–2003), whom he divorced in 1977. Towards the end of his life he was in a relationship with Françoise Kestsman, a local woman, who was his secretary, housekeeper and lover until his death.

Claude devoted herself to Durrell. The fact she was married with two children when meeting Durrell is underplayed in all his biographies. According to MacNiven, in a private correspondence with me, Claude in fact abandoned her children for her relationship with Durrell. In the course of their ten years together, she met them only on their summer holidays from the boarding schools they attended. She decided to sacrifice the presence of her children in her life for her relationship with Durrell. She arranged for them to attend prestigious boarding schools and left most of the parental care to their father, whom she divorced. In her posthumously published diaries, Sappho Durrell mentions Claude's children on several occasions and describes their summer encounters as exciting, while also citing the emotional difficulties the two had every time they had to part from their mother. The prospect of them living with Durrell and Claude was never realised, apart from holiday visits. Sappho herself puts it down to Claude's refusal to reckon with the emotional complexity that this arrangement would entail for her.

The tale of Durrell's "ten good years," which saw him writing his most significant and accomplished work, has a different angle therefore if we add to it the narrative of Claude's children. Their mother's decision to leave her children and pursue a life of writing alongside Durrell, first in Cyprus then in the south of France, came at a cost. In their book on the crisis of witnessing in literature, Felman and Laub write:

> Biography and history are neither simply represented nor simply reflected, but are reinscribed, translated, radically rethought and fundamentally worked over by the text. In order to gain insight into the significance and impact of the context on the text, the empirical context needs not just to be *known*, but to be *read*; to be read in conjunction with, and as part of, the reading of the text. We thus propose to show how the basic and legitimate critical demand for *contextualization of the text* itself needs to be complemented, simultaneously, by the less familiar and yet necessary work of *textualization of the context*.[89]

The major *text* in this case is the tale of the *ten happy years*, while the latent *context* is the cost exacted by this success story on the lost, crossed-out witnesses, the children of Claude. The testimony of her children has never been written down or never told in a manner that left any traces. Sappho described Durrell's relationships in the years that followed Claude's death as gloomy. In her eyes too, the stability that marked Durrell's life in his years with Claude, when Sappho herself found a cosy home in the south of France, fell apart with Claude's death. She could not bear to be in touch with her father, now that he was alone. His emotional aggression towards his nearest and dearest women became intolerable. "Trying to think why my relationship with my father is now so fucked up. I used to write him letters, but since Claude died his traditional pattern of wife=whore/stupid/bitch and me=virgin/wise has disintegrated."[90]

The posthumous publication of Sappho's selected journals and letters in 1991 created a major controversy among the literary and academic Durrellian community.[91] It was claimed that the publication of Sappho's diaries featured evidence that Durrell had had sexual relations with his daughter following Claude's death, when Sappho had been sixteen.[92] As Sappho and Durrell were dead by the time of these allegations, they remained hypothetical. These allegations were unanimously rejected by Durrell's living relatives, including his brother Gerald, his sister Margaret and his ex-wives Nancy and Eve.[93] In his 2009 review of a new book that rekindled discussion into these allegations, James Gifford wrote that there was enough evidence to show that Durrell's relationship with his daughter had been fraught even without substantiating those allegations, which could be neither confirmed no refuted.[94] Gordon Bowker, author of Durrell's critical biography, also assumes that there is no way either to prove or disprove these allegations. According to him, Durrell's pervasive involvement in his daughter's life following Claude's death meant a heavy emotional burden for Sappho, which left evident traces in her diaries and letters. Bowker believes that the *Sunday Times* story by Barbara Robson was part of that period's trend of dredging up repressed childhood memories.[95] Sappho's diaries and letters portray an image of life in the Durrell household more than a decade after Claude's death. The excerpts from the diaries and letters date back to 1979, the year when Sappho embarked on psychoanalysis with Patrick Casement in London.[96] At the time, she was living away from her father, yet kept in touch with regular visits every couple of months. Sappho wrote from a perspective of more than a decade after Claude's death. Therapy perhaps allowed her to take an unflinching look deep down into her psychic experiences, where her father featured prominently. Her journals of that period are replete with details of her childhood following her weekly analysis sessions with Casement. She takes a meticulous account of the number of monthly appointments and their fees. She describes the childhood of her mother and father as told to her and the emotionally violent relationships between her parents and recalls the night they broke up following a loud row.[97] The story she portrays is a sad one, culminating in her own desperation and eventual suicide.

Death

On October 1978, twelve years prior to his own death, Durrell wrote a revealing letter to Miller, its tone anguished though resigned to his condition:

> Yes, I am living alone. IT'S WONDERFUL. I have to answer to nobody; sometimes a nymph strays into my net – I keep all the twigs limed, mind you. . . . But I have at last got on top of that terrible hippogriff – "unable to be alone"; in the course of this whole evolution I have learnt to cook for myself and clean for myself. No sailor can match me now. . . . The autumn is big and heavy and the wine is safely in; the days boom like an empty barrel and the insects fly slowly about, half dead with ripeness.[98]

These words are the words of an old man who is resigned to his fate. He describes loneliness as a developmental accomplishment, as he has finally learnt to live on his own, despite the fact that he was to spend the last years of his life in the company of the loving and caring Françoise Kestsman whom he nearly married.

The author of *The Alexandria Quartet* had found his lost homeland in his work. In his individuality, he reverted to the same primeval state to which he had striven in the reflective process of writing. It is Durrell's original aloof position, which he expressed in the concept of *the Heraldic Universe*.[99] Durrell is one of a kind. By his own assertion, he is of a different breed. His affinity remained ambivalent. His endeavour of re-finding his homeland took him on a marvellous journey of writing, where he explored his life and made sense of it. However, he remained alone in his *unheimliche* universe of his own making. His glaring individuality leaves him alone on the desert island of his existence in his turbulent and rich universe, entire of itself. He left us his words to be inspired by in our own quest for meaning.

Notes

1 Kristeva, Julia, 1991, *Strangers to Ourselves*, trans. L. S. Roudiez, New York: Columbia University Press, p. 5.
2 Nin, Anaïs, 1967, *The Journals of Anaïs Nin, Vol. Six 1955–1966*, London: Quartet Books, p. 125.
3 MacNiven, Ian S., 1998, *Lawrence Durrell: A Biography*, London: Faber & Faber, p. 187.
4 Durrell, Lawrence, 1983, "Interview with Piero Sanavio", in *La Stampa*, pp. 21–26. Durrell also wrote of D. H. Lawrence in the *Quartet*'s fourth volume, *Clea*, when ascribing one of the protagonists, Pursewarden, a close friendship with the writer (Durrell, Lawrence, 1960, *Clea*, London: Faber & Faber, p. 141).
5 Dearborn, Mary V., 1991, *The Happiest Man Alive: A Biography of Henry Miller*, New York: Simon & Schuster.
6 Miller, Henry, 1934, *Tropic of Cancer*, New York: Grove Press.
7 Miller, Henry, 1949, *Sexus*, New York: Grove Press.
8 Ingersoll, Earl G., 1998, *Lawrence Durrell: Conversations*, London: Associated University Presses, pp. 12–34.
9 Durrell, Lawrence, 1980b, *A Smile in the Mind's Eye*, London: Wildwood House, p. 18.
10 Durrell, Lawrence, 1957a, *Justine*, London: Faber & Faber, pp. 159–160.
11 Richard Pine has referred to the Primal Wound when he described Durrell's lifelong struggle for his lost fragment. According to Pine's interpretation of Durrell's own words, that wound was caused by his birth experience and his sense of lost childhood. Pine, Richard, 2005, *Lawrence Durrell: The Mindscape*, Corfu: Durrell School of Corfu, pp. 83–84.
12 MacNiven, Ian S., 1998, *Lawrence Durrell: A Biography*, London: Faber & Faber.
13 Bowker, Gordon, 1997, *Through the Dark Labyrinth: A Biography of Lawrence Durrell*, London: St. Martin's Press.
14 Pine, Richard, 2005, *Lawrence Durrell: The Mindscape*, Corfu: The Durrell School of Corfu. The Durrell School of Corfu was founded by Pine in 2001. It was closed in 2014 and reopened in 2016 under a new name, The Durrell Library of Corfu.
15 Botting, Douglas, 1999, *Gerald Durrell: The Authorized Biography*, New York: Carrol & Graf.
16 MacNiven, Ian S., ed. 1988, *The Durrell-Miller Letters, 1935–1980*, London: Faber & Faber.
17 MacNiven, Ian S. and Harry T. Moore, eds. 1981, *Literary Lifelines, the Richard Aldington: Lawrence Durrell Correspondence*, London: Faber & Faber. There are several other letter collections which I have not drawn from in this study such as the correspondence with the Greek poet and doctor Theodore Stephanides (1896–1983), whom Durrell met in 1935, the French poet and psychoanalyst Jean Fanchette (1932–1992) and the American poet Gostan [Kostan] Zarian (1885–1969), all of whom were significant to Durrell at various points in his life.
18 Durrell, Sappho, 1991, "Journals and Letters", in *The Family: They Fuck You Up*, London: Granta.
19 Nin, Anaïs, 1966, *The Journals of Anaïs Nin, Vol. Two 1934–1939*, London: Quartet Books; Nin, Anaïs, 1967, *The Journals of Anaïs Nin, Vol. Six 1955–1966*, London: Quartet Books; Nin Anaïs, 1980, *The Journals of Anaïs Nin, Vol. Seven 1966–1974*, London: Quartet Books; Miller, Henry, 1952, *The Books in My Life*, London: Viking Press.

20 Unterecker, John, 1964, *Lawrence Durrell*, New York and London: Columbia University Press.
21 Weigel, John A., 1965, *Lawrence Durrell*, New York: Twayne Publishers Inc.
22 Kipling, Rudyard, 1993, *Kim*, Hertfordshire: Wordsworth Editions Limited.
23 Durrell, Lawrence, 1969, *Spirit of Place: Letters and Essays on Travel*, ed. Alan G. Thomas, Mount Jackson: Axios Press, p. 50.
24 MacNiven, Ian S., 1998, *Lawrence Durrell: A Biography*, London: Faber & Faber, p. 14.
25 Durrell, Lawrence, 1980b, *A Smile in the Mind's Eye*, London: Wildwood House, p. 50.
26 Durrell, Sappho, 1991, "Journals and Letters", in *The Family: They Fuck You Up*, London: Granta, p. 61.
27 Rank, Otto, 1932, *The Myth of the Birth of the Hero*, trans. Gregory C. Richter and E. James Lieberman, New York: Vintage Books, p. 193.
28 MacNiven, Ian S., 1998, *Lawrence Durrell: A Biography*, London: Faber & Faber, p. 17.
29 Bowker, Gordon, 1997, *Through the Dark Labyrinth: A Biography of Lawrence Durrell*, London: St. Martin's Press, p. 9.
30 Durrell offered a vividly Kiplingian account of this disease, true to his view that his life in India was a personal variation on Kipling's *Kim*. He claimed to have remembered the various efforts of his Indian nannies to boost his failing health as a baby with cobra blood potion and walks around the local cemetery. He even remembered, apparently, coming upon carrions picked at by birds of prey and hyenas.
31 Durrell, Sappho, 1991, "Journals and Letters", in *The Family: They Fuck You Up*, London: Granta, pp. 62–65.
32 MacNiven, Ian S., ed. 1988, *The Durrell-Miller Letters, 1935–1980*, London: Faber & Faber, p. 321.
33 Botting, Douglas, 1999, *Gerald Durrell: The Authorized Biography*, New York: Carrol & Graf, pp. 3–8.
34 MacNiven, Ian, S., 2000, "Margaret Durrell Remembers . . .", *Deus Loci*, 8:3–25.
35 Durrell, Gerald, 2016 (1956), *My Family and Other Animal*, London: Macmillan Collector's Library, p. 10.
36 Weigel, John A., 1965, *Lawrence Durrell*, New York: Twayne Publishers Inc., p. 19.
37 Pine, Richard, 2005, *Lawrence Durrell: The Mindscape*, Corfu: Durrell School of Corfu, p. 42.
38 MacNiven too assumed that the Indian uprising led by Mahatma Gandhi made Lawrence Samuel fear instability (MacNiven, Ian S., 1998, *Lawrence Durrell: A Biography*, London: Faber & Faber, p. 24).
39 MacNiven, Ian S., 1998, *Lawrence Durrell: A Biography*, London: Faber & Faber, p. 29.
40 Henty, George, 2015, *The Lion of St. Mark*, London: Lulu.com.
41 Durrell was particularly inspired by Haggard's *King Solomon's Mines* (Haggard, H. Rider, 1994, King Solomon's Mines, London: Penguin Books), which was also a formative experience for Henry Miller. Miller too wrote about his experience of reading this book: Miller, Henry, 1952, *The Books in My Life*, London: Viking Press, pp. 81–100.
42 Durrell, Lawrence, 1957b, *Bitter Lemons*, London: Fabre & Faber, p. 67.
43 MacNiven, Ian S., 1998, *Lawrence Durrell: A Biography*, London: Faber & Faber, p. 29.
44 Alice Miller (1923–2010), a Swiss psychoanalyst, wrote several books regarding what she termed as *poisonous pedagogy* by which she referred to various child-rearing practices, such as sending boys away from home, that were customary amongst certain classes and only later were seen to be damaging to the well-being of the children. Miller, Alice, 1987, *The Drama of Being a Child*, London: Virago Books.
45 One of his classmates was Abba Eben (1915–2002), the Foreign Minister of Israel 1966–1974.
46 Durrell, Lawrence, 1958b, *Mountolive*, London: Faber & Faber, p. 22.
47 MacNiven, Ian S., 1998, *Lawrence Durrell: A Biography*, London: Faber & Faber, pp. 47–49.
48 Ibid., p. 42.
49 Bowker, Gordon, 1997, *Through the Dark Labyrinth: A Biography of Lawrence Durrell*, London: St. Martin's Press, pp. 19–39, 424–437.

50 Durrell, Sappho, 1991, "Journals and Letters", in *The Family: They Fuck You Up*, London: Granta, pp. 69–70.
51 Dibdin, Michael, 1990, "One Man's Retreat from Pudding Island", *Independent on Sunday*, November 11, p. 27.
52 Durrell, Lawrence, 1958a, *Balthazar*, London: Faber & Faber, p. 65.
53 Durrell's father, as noted before, chose the timing of his son's banishment with care. He feared that if he stayed in India beyond the age of eleven, he would fail to master the "right" British accent and be stamped with the lilting local accent that would forever set him apart from his desired class. His zealous pursuit of the "right accent" reflected, among other things, in his insistence that the local servants hold all their communications with the children strictly in Hindi, so as not to expose them to the local English accent.
54 Durrell, Lawrence, 1958b, *Mountolive*, London: Faber & Faber, p. 97.
55 Durrell, Sappho, 1991, "Journals and Letters", in *The Family: They Fuck You Up*, London: Granta, p. 71.
56 MacNiven, Ian S., 1998, *Lawrence Durrell: A Biography*, London: Faber & Faber, p. 68.
57 The full term is a failed BA of Benares University.
58 Durrell, Lawrence, 1958b, *Mountolive*, London: Faber & Faber, p. 104.
59 Bowker, Gordon, 1997, *Through the Dark Labyrinth: A Biography of Lawrence Durrell*, London: St. Martin's Press, p. 8.
60 MacNiven, Ian S., 1998, *Lawrence Durrell: A Biography*, London: Faber & Faber, p. 65.
61 Ibid., p. 18.
62 MacNiven, Ian S., 1998, *Lawrence Durrell: A Biography*, London: Faber & Faber, p. 106.
63 It was finally published by Faber & Faber in 1973. In 1937 Faber & Faber had published an earlier novel Durrell had written, *Panic Spring*, under the pseudonym Charles Norden, as the very first novel Durrell published by Cassell in 1935, *Piped Piper of Lovers*, did not succeed commercially. Before *The Black Book* had achieved the critical acclaim that it had, Durrell seriously considered conducting two parallel literary careers: one as himself and another as Charles Norden. For further reading, see Richard Pine, 2018, "Lawrence Durrell's Minor Mythologies" in his *Minor Mythologies as Popular Literature*, Cambridge: Cambridge Scholars Publishing.
64 The Greek word agon can be understood in several ways. As well as describing an athletic contest, it also means a struggle and can be seen in its later developments in words as Prot*agon*ist and *agony*. I suggest that Durrell used the word in its full, multiple implications.
65 Durrell, Lawrence, 1938, *The Black Book*, London: Faber & Faber, p. 20.
66 It was those explicit accounts that meant that the book was banned for publication in England for many years. It was only openly distributed during the late 1950s.
67 Durrell, Lawrence, 1938, *The Black Book*, London: Faber & Faber, p. 22.
68 These excerpts are from a string of letters he wrote to his friend, Alan G. Thomas (1911–1992). Durrell, Lawrence, 1969, *Spirit of Place: Letters and Essays on Travel*, ed. Alan G. Thomas, Mount Jackson: Axios Press, pp. 33–61.
69 Ibid., pp. 49–50.
70 Ibid., p. 60.
71 Ibid., pp. 61–62.
72 Bloom, Harold, 1973, *The Anxiety of Influence*, Oxford: Oxford University Press, p. 70.
73 For full detailed exploration of the diverse literary influences upon Durrell's writing, a field I will not explore further in this study, the best source is Pine, Richard, 2005, *Lawrence Durrell: The Mindscape*, Corfu: Durrell School of Corfu.
74 MacNiven, Ian S., ed. 1988, *The Durrell-Miller Letters, 1935–1980*, London: Faber & Faber, p. 21.
75 Miller, Henry, 1934, *Tropic of Cancer*, New York: Grove Press, p. 5.
76 Durrell, Lawrence, 1938, *The Black Book*, London: Faber & Faber, p. 20.
77 Durrell, Lawrence, 1969, *Spirit of Place*, ed. Alan T. Thomas, Mount Jackson: Axios Press, p. 79.
78 MacNiven, Ian S., ed. 1988, *The Durrell-Miller Letters, 1935–1980*, London: Faber & Faber, p. 144.

79 In this capacity Durrell was put in charge of newspapers in the three languages distributed in Cyprus, as well as several radio stations, speaking several languages, and coordinated various cultural activities. As part of his high-ranking position, Durrell rubbed shoulders with many local politicians and so, in 1957, as riots broke out on the island, he had to leave due to fears for his life.

80 Claude conducted her liaison with Durrell while still married. Several months after Durrell and she moved in together, her husband made a surprise visit to Cyprus. Durrell and Claude tried to keep their relationship secret from him, but as it became public, it did not provoke her husband's wrath. The couple divorced about a year later, but their children stayed in boarding schools and spent their holidays with Durrell and their mother in France.

81 Nin, Anäis, 1967, *The Journals of Anäis Nin, Vol. Six 1955–1966*, London: Quartet Books, p. 107.

82 Claude's first novel, entitled *Mrs. O*, was published in 1957. She published two additional books, *The Rum* Go (1958) and *A Chair for the Prophet* (1959), its plot set in Israel.

83 Nin, Anaïs, 1980, *The Journals of Anaïs Nin, Vol. Seven 1966–1974*, London: Quartet Books, p. 297.

84 MacNiven, Ian S., 1998, *Lawrence Durrell: A Biography*, London: Faber & Faber, p. 645.

85 Haag, Michael, 2004, *Alexandria, City of Memory*, London: Yale University Press, pp. 318–330.

86 The *Lavon Affair* was an abortive Israeli covert operation conducted in Egypt in 1954, involving local Egyptian Jews, aimed to place several bombs in key locations and to blame an extremist Muslim group in doing so, and thus provoke the British government to keep its armed forces in the Suez Canal area. The operation was not carried through and the only casualties were four operatives who were captured. Two of them killed themselves and the other two were tried and executed. The Israeli Defense Minister at the time, Pinchas Lavon (1904–1972), was forced to resign when the details of the failed operation came out.

87 MacNiven, Ian S., ed. 1988, *The Durrell-Miller Letters, 1935–1980*, London: Faber & Faber, p. 361.

88 Ibid., pp. 418–442.

89 Felman, Shoshana and Laub Dori, 1992, *Testimony: Crises of Witnessing in Literature, Psychoanalysis and History*, London & New York: Routledge, p. 59.

90 Durrell, Sappho, 1991, "Journals and Letters", in *The Family: They Fuck You Up*, London: Granta, p. 61.

91 Robson, Barbara, 1991, "The Darker Side of Durrell", *The Sunday Telegraph*, May 26, pp. 23–26.

92 Durrell, Sappho, 1991, "Journals and Letters", in *The Family: They Fuck You Up*, London: Granta, pp. 55–92.

93 Botting, Douglas, 1999, *Gerald Durrell: The Authorized Biography*, New York: Carrol & Graf, pp. 565–566.

94 Gifford, James, 2009, "Incest: A New Perspective", *Deus Loci*, 11:133–139.

95 Bowker, Gordon, 1997, *Through the Dark Labyrinth: A Biography of Lawrence Durrell*, London: St. Martin's Press, pp. 428–430.

96 Patrick Casement is a British psychoanalyst and social worker who gained renown in the 1980s following the publication of his book *On Learning from the Patient* (1985). The book expounds the insights gained from his clinical experience regarding the importance of paying attention to his occasional mistakes as analyst when reading the patient. According to him, attention to, and learning from, these mistakes allow a more ethical therapeutic process and pave the way for mental change, for the analyst and patient alike.

97 Bowker, Gordon, 1997, *Through the Dark Labyrinth: A Biography of Lawrence Durrell*, London: St. Martin's Press, p. 69.

98 MacNiven, Ian S., ed. 1988, *The Durrell-Miller Letters, 1935–1980*, London: Faber & Faber, pp. 497–498.

99 Durrell, Lawrence, 1969, *Spirit of Place: Letters and Essays on Travel*, ed. Alan G. Thomas, Mount Jackson: Axios Press, pp. 61–62.

6
EPILOGUE

This book studies Lawrence Durrell's endeavour to deal with his experience of *das unheimliche* The Uncanny through his writing and to establish his inner world as a place he could call his home. His personal circumstances made him perceive himself as a solitary being looking out on the world from his aloof and distant position. Such an experience of solitude made him emphasise the endeavours of the individual towards self-fulfilment when his environment was experienced as alien and often inferior. He drew inspiration from his surrounding, but did not always fully acknowledge its immense value in constituting his identity as a writer.

The *Quartet* served as a transitional and liminal *unheimliche* home-space for the author where he shaped the different aspects of his belonging to his imaginary homeland. The interpretation of the *Quartet* shows how the interweaving of its biographical and fictional elements charts the author's reflective process as he wrote the tetralogy. This study rests on three conceptual nodal points: the biographical-fictional binary in the interpretation of literary works, the convergence of psychoanalysis and literature and the concepts of belonging and exile.

The *Quartet* is by no means unintelligible and does not need a theoretical interpretation to make sense it. This study is an encounter between two languages, two cultures: that of the words written by Durrell and those written by a few psychoanalytic thinkers. It is a journey in both the worlds of the *Quartet* and of psychoanalysis, a reading, encountering and ingesting of texts so as to make them into a live presence.

Previous studies have critically contrasted psychoanalytic studies of literature with interpretations of the literary text outside its context. The hermeneutic outlook of the present study is that the biographical and fictional elements are a single whole which yields the major questions that emerge from the text. The enterprise of clarifying the biographical aspects and their relation to the fictional elements in a work of literature is not about reducing the text to a psychological account; it is about showing the affinity of the text with the life of the author, as well as their mutually exerted influence and how they are reflected in the text itself.

This monograph studies the complex issue of the individual sense of belonging to his homeland and how this belonging is reflected in the act of writing. This sense can be best summarised through the Freudian use of the term *das unheimliche* – the strangeness of the homely – the *Uncanny*. One's home is both the safe place where the individual can create and at the very same time also the one place which endangers his freedom. It is this paradoxical nature of the homeland, and of relationships, which strikes the key note throughput this psychoanalytic study of the *Quartet*.

The author of the tetralogy, Lawrence Durrell, is not an "ordinary" exile in its strict sense. When writing *The Alexandria Quartet* he modelled the work as his imaginary homeland. It was in this work that Durrell expressed the complexity of his belonging experience and reflected upon his life. The fragmentary nature of the tetralogy, with its multiple narrative voices and intricate, contradictory plotlines, allowed him to express different biographical aspects of his life. Durrell's exile stemmed from his compromised childhood experience, his *secret wound*. The undermining of the primeval, Edenic experience, formed the hotbed for the reflective process to evolve through writing, a process that allowed him to try to return, through a *return of the repressed* to a sense of his lost self.

This *return*, the topography of the work, rests on two organising principles. The first principle is reliance on modern theories of the time and space perception. The second one is a complex, multi-layered perception of the narrator, who is in fact a multiple voice. The time perception in this work differentiates between historical time and subjective time. The inspiration for this differentiation is Albert Einstein's theory of relativity, showing that the perception of reality is subjective. The characters of this work hold different, at times opposing, perceptions regarding the same event. These complexities are inspired by psychoanalytical concepts that Durrell was influenced by, which differentiate between conscious and unconscious parts of the mind. The entire work was constructed as a metaphor of the author's mind, which cannot be identified with any single character, but rather with a whole gamut of voices that come together to form a whole mind that is "responsible" for the entire work.

The multiplicity of the narrative voices, and the blurred boundaries between them and the protagonists, suggests that the *unheimliche* homeland that is *The Alexandria Quartet* can be termed as a *poetic space* – which is no mere concrete and geographical description, but a space that retains human passions and dreams. The entire work is a dynamic entity that metamorphoses according to the different positions taken by the different characters.

The author's prefatory notes to the four single volumes edition, and the workpoints that conclude three of them, constitute the setting of the work. Beyond the topographical demarcation that these constitute for the body of the work, they reflect the author's reflective process. Psychoanalytic ideas inspired Lawrence Durrell in his writing of *The Alexandria Quartet*, which is particularly evident in his use of dreams. Freud described the dream as the highway to the unconsciousness. The focus on dreams reflected therefore part of the author's reflective process.

At the heart of this work lies the *poetic space* occupied by the *mother-city* of Alexandria. This space is where the narrative voices express their reflective process. It is described as a sexual and maternal omnipotent being, an unconscious force that decides her people's fate, as they have little control over it. Three perspectives were employed to show this. The first perspective concerned the author's *Weltanschauung*, with its inherent contradiction that pits the individual's quest for self-fulfilment against his belonging to broader setting and tradition. The second perspective pertained to the city's perception as at once a biographical and fictional entity. His experiences in the city formed the bedrock from which *The Alexandria Quartet's* materials were taken, though written more than a decade after he had left the city. The third and main perspective concerned the multiple characterisations of Alexandria as the *mother-city* against which inner and interpersonal drama play out.

The author's quest to make sense of his existence in the liminal space of the poetic city is an expression of *the Heraldic Universe*. Perhaps a too clear definition of this idiosyncratic original Durrellian term will spoil its charm. It is perhaps best to think of it as a poetic expression of what Durrell held most dear in his life. Like a poem, it is advised to allow its magic to work without taking it apart to examine its workings. Still, it might be safe to say that Durrell tried to signify the solitude of the individual and the ultimate value of self-expression as a value that cannot be surpassed. Durrell introduces *the Heraldic Universe* as a spiritual symbol of the individual aspiration for fulfilment and the realisation of his inner vision. For all his efforts to expand his consciousness and engage his surroundings in such a way that would not compromise their differentiation and independence, he remains an aloof figure, detached from life and preoccupied with the compulsive return to writing, the only daily act where he could find expression and meaning. The author's interest in his surroundings and people is part of his inner drama.

The characters in the tetralogy abide by rules and imperatives that are seemingly beyond their control. They try to break through by engaging in perverse sexuality to achieve liberation and salvation, and time and again end up getting wounded by their own efforts. The individual quest for his identity is relentless, despite his growing recognition that this search is doomed to fail. The failure also belies hope, for the search itself, the reflective process evoked by the act of writing, is in fact the purpose. Self-knowledge, the purpose of the reflective process, is underpinned by an element of hope. This is not an aspiration for transcendental truth, as truth cannot be a single, unequivocal entity as long as language mediates its utterance. The nature of language allows transforming reality into art and art into reality, and it is there that hope lies for the realisation of man's aspiration for self-discovery.

The Alexandria Quartet uniquely conveys the author's aim of showing that his reflective process is designed for the purpose of making sense of life. Durrell wrote because without writing he felt alienation and failed to make sense of his life. Writing served as his vital channel for expression, while writing this work in particular represented for him the home he had aspired to return to throughout his life.

BIBLIOGRAPHY

Alexandre-Garner, Corinne, 1997, "The Enigma of the *Quartet*", in Robert Ilbert, ed., *Alexandria 1960–1980: The Brief Life of a Cosmopolitan Community*, Alexandria: Harpocrete Publishing, pp. 162–167.

Adam, Peter, 1987, "Alexandria Revisited", in *Twentieth Century Revisited, 33/3:* 395–410.

———, 1998, "Everything Comes Right", in Earl Ingersoll, ed., *Lawrence Durrell: Conversations*, Cranbury, NJ: Associated University Presses, pp. 163–170.

Alfandary, Rony, 2016, "To Write or Not to Write: Is That the Question?" A Therapeutic Tale (Hebrew) *Maárg*, 7:1–18.

———, 2016, ed., *Seeking Psychic Space: Fundamentals of Psychodynamic Social Work (Hebrew)*, Jerusalem: Carmel Publishers.

Armstrong, James, 1996, "Banned in America by the U.S. Customs Officials", in *Bibliographical Society of America*, 34:230–256.

Azoulay, Ariella, 2007, *Once Upon a Time: Photography Following Walter Benjamin (Hebrew).* Ramat-Gan: Bar-Ilan University Press.

Bachelard, Gaston, 1994, *The Poetics of Space*, trans. Maria Jolas, Boston: Beacon Press.

Bakhtin, Michail, 1986, "From Notes Made in 1970–1971", in *Speech Genres & Other Late Essays*, trans. V. Mcgee, Texas: University of Texas Press.

Barchilon, Jose, 1971, "A Study of Camus' Mythpoeic Tale *the Fall* with Some Comments About the Origin of Esthetic Feelings", *Journal of American Psychoanalysis Association*, 19:193–240.

Barthes, Roland, 1972, *Mythologies*, trans. Annette Lavers, New York: The Noonday Press.

———, 1977, "Death of the Author", in *Image, Music, Text*, trans. Stephen Heath, London: Fontana Press.

Bauman, Zygmunt, 1990, "Modernity and Ambivalence", in Featherstone Mike, ed., *Global Culture: Nationalism, Globalization and Modernity*, London: Sage.

———, 2003, *Liquid Love*, Cambridge: Polity Press.

Begnal, Michael H., 1990, *On Miracle Ground*, London: Associated University Press.

Belfer, Ella, 2004, *A Split Identity: The Conflict between the Sacred and the Secular in the Jewish World (Hebrew)*, Ramta-Gan: Bar-Ilan University Press.

Berman, Emanuel, ed., 1993, *Essential Papers on Literature and Psychoanalysis*, New York and London: New York University Press.

Bertin, Celia, 1983, *Marie Bonaparte: A Life,* London: Quartet Books.

Bhabha, Homi, 1992, "The World and the Home", *Social Text*, 31/32:141–152.

———, 1994, *The Location of Culture*, London & New York: Routledge.

Bion, Wilfred R., 1963, *Elements of Psycho-Analysis*, London: Maresfield and Karnac Books.

Bloom, Harold, 1997, *The Anxiety of Influence*, New York and Oxford: Oxford University Press.

———, 2005, *Julio Cortázar*, Philadelphia: Chelsea House Publications, pp. 87–90.

Boccia, Michael, 1989, "Lawrence Durrell's *Alexandria Quartet*: Novel and Palimpsest", in *Form as Content and Rhetoric in the Modern Novel*, New York: Peter Lang, pp. 149–181.

Bode, Carl, 1961, "Durrell's Way to Alexandria", *College English*, 22/8:531–538.

Bollas, Christopher, 1987, *The Shadow of the Object*, London: Free Association Books.

———, 1991, *Forces of Destiny*, London: Free Association Books.

———, 2007, *The Freudian Moment*, London: Karnac Books.

Bonaparte, Marie, 1935, "The Murders in Rue Morgue", *The Psychonalytic Quarterly*, 4:259–293.

Boone, Joseph Allen, 1998, "Fifties Writing Gone Mad", in *Libidinal Currents: Sexuality and the Shaping of Modernity*, Chicago: University of Chicago Press, pp. 253–276.

Bork, Alfred, 1963, "Durell and Relativity", *The Centennial Review*, 16:191–203.

Botting, Douglas, 1999, *Gerald Durrell: The Authorized Biography*, New York: Carrol & Graff.

Bowker, Gordon, 1997, *Through the Dark Labyrinth: A Biography of Lawrence Durrell*, London: St. Martin's Press.

Brassaï, 1995, *Henry Miller: The Paris Years*, New York: Arcade Publishing, pp. 199–205.

Brewster, Chamerberlin, 2007, *Lawrence Durrell Chronology*, Corfu: Durrell School of Corfu.

Brink, Andrew, 1977, *Loss and Symbolic Repair: A Psychological Study of Some English Poets*, Ontario: The Cromlech Press.

Cavafy, C. P., 1992, *Collected Poems*, ed., George Savidis, trans. Edmund Keeley and Philip Sherrard, Revised Edition, Princeton, NJ: Princeton University Press.

Casement, Patrick, 1990, *Learning from the Patient*, New York: The Guilford Press.

Chasseuegt-Smirgel, Janine, 1984, *Creativity and Perversion*, London: Free Association Books.

Cleyet, George, 1980, "The Villa Seurat Circle: Creative Nexus", *Deus Loci*, 4:4–6.

Colas, Santiago, 2005, "Inventing Autonomies, Meditations on Julio Cortázar and the Politics of Our Time", *The New Centennial Review*, 5/2:1–34.

Cortázar, Julio, 1966, *Hopscotch*, trans. Gregory Rabassa, New York: Pantheon Books.

Dawson, Carl, 1970, "From Einstein to Keats", *Far Eastern Forum*, 1:109–127.

De Sade, Marquis, 2008, *Justine or 'Good Conduct Well Chastised'*, Radford: Wilder Publications.

Dearborn, Mary V., 1991, *The Happiest Man Alive: A Biography of Henry Miller*, New York: Simon & Schuster.

Deep, Marquis, 1991, "Mahfouz and Durrell", in Gassick Trevor, ed., in *Critical Views on Naguib Mahfouz*, Washington, DC: Three Continents, pp. 27–37.

Derrida, Jacques, 2000, *On Hospitality*, trans. Rachel Bowlby, Stanford: Stanford University Press.

Diboll, Mike, 2004, *Lawrence Durrell's Alexandria Quartet in Its Egyptian Context*, London: Edwin Mellen Press Ltd.

Durrell, Gerald, 1956 (2016), *My Family and Other Animals*, London: Macmillan Collector's Library.

Durrell, Lawrence, 1935, *Pied Piper of Lovers*, London: Cassell & Co.

———, 1937, *Panic Spring: A Romance*, London: Faber & Faber.

———, 1938, *The Black Book: An Agon*, Villa Seurat Series 1, Paris: Obelisk Press.

———, 1939, "Hamlet, Prince of China", in *Delta*, 23:38–45.

———, 1945, *Prospero's Cell: A Guide to the Landscape and Manners of the Island of Corcyra*, London: Faber & Faber.

———, 1946, "Introduction", in *E.M. Forster's Alexandria: History and Guide*, New York: Oxford University Press.
———, 1947a, *The Dark Labyrinth*, London: Faber & Faber.
———, 1947b, "Can Dreams Live on when Dreamers Die?" *The Listener*, September 25.
———, 1952a, *A Key to Modern British Poetry*, London: Peter Neville.
———, 1952b, *Sappho*, London: Faber & Faber.
———, 1957a, *Justine*, London: Faber & Faber.
———, 1957b, *Bitter Lemons*, London: Faber & Faber.
———, 1958a, *Balthazar*, London: Faber & Faber.
———, 1958b, *Mountolive*, London: Faber & Faber.
———, 1959, *Alfred Perlès, and Henry Miller, Art and Outrage: A Correspondence about Henry Miller between Alfred Perlès and Lawrence Durrell*, London: Putnam.
———, 1960, *Clea*, London: Faber & Faber.
———, 1961, "Introduction", in *The Book of the It, Georg Groddeck*, London: Vision Press, pp. 34–78.
———, 1962, *The Alexandria Quartet*, London: Faber & Faber.
———, 1968, *Tunc*, London: Faber & Faber.
———, 1969, *Spirit of Place: Letters and Essays on Travel*, ed. Alan G. Thomas, Mount Jackson: Axios Press.
———, 1970, *Nunquam*, London: Faber & Faber.
———, 1974a, *Monsieur, or The Prince of Darkness*, London: Faber & Faber.
———, 1974b, *The Best of Antrobus*, London: Faber & Faber.
———, 1974c, *The Revolt of Aphrodite*, London: Faber & Faber.
———, 1978a, *The Greek Islands*, London: Faber & Faber.
———, 1978b, *Livia, or Buried Alive*, London: Faber & Faber.
———, 1980a, *Collected Poems, 1931–1974*, ed. James A. Brigham. London: Faber & Faber.
———, 1980b, *A Smile in the Mind's Eye*, London: Wildwood House.
———, 1982, *Constance, or Solitary Practices*, London: Faber & Faber.
———, 1983, *Sebastian, or Ruling Passions*, London: Faber & Faber.
———, 1985, *Quinx, or The Ripper's Tale*, London: Faber & Faber.
———, 1987, "Letters to T. S. Eliot" in *Twentieth Century Literature*, 33/3:348–358.
———, 1990, *Caesar's Vast Ghost*, London: Faber & Faber.
———, 2004, *The Lawrence Durrell Travel Reader*, ed. Clint Willis. New York: Carroll & Graf.
———, 2012, *Judith*, Corfu: Durrell School of Corfu.
———, 2015, *From the Elephant's back: Collected Essays & Travel Writings*, Gifford, James, ed., Edmonton: The University of Alberta Press.
———, 2018a, *The Placebo*, ed. Richard Pine and David Roessel, London: Colenso Books.
———, 2018b, *The Fruitful Discontent of the World: a further collection of poems by Lawrence Durrell*, London: Colenso Books and the Delos Press.
Durrell, Sappho, 1991, "Journals and Letters", in *The Family: They Fuck You Up*, London: Granta, pp. 55–92.
Eagleton, Terry, 1998, "Supreme Trickster", *The New Statesman*, April 24, pp. 48–49.
Eskin, Stanley, 1962, "Durrell's Themes in *The Alexandria Quartet*", *Texas Quarterly*, Winter: 43–60.
Felman, Shoshana, 1977, *Literature and Psychoanalysis*, Baltimore and London: The John Hopkins University Press.
———, 2003, *Writing and Madness*, Palo Alto: Stanford University Press.
Felman, Shoshana and Laub, Dori, 1992, *Testimony: Crises of Witnessing in Literature, Psychoanalysis, and History*, London & New York: Routledge.

Festa-McCormick, Diana, 1979, "Durrell's *Alexandria Quartet*: A Whore Amongst Cities", in *The City as Catalyst: A Study of Ten Novels*, Cranbury, NJ: Associated Universities Presses, pp. 158–176.

Forster, E. M., 1961, *Alexandria: History and Guide*, New York: Doubleday.

Franklin, Steve, 1979, "Space-Time and Creativity in Lawrence Durrell's the *Alexandria Quartet*", *Perspectives on Modern Literature*, 5:55–61.

Fraser, G. S., 1968, *Lawrence Durrell*, London: Faber & Faber.

Freud, Sigmund, 1899, "Screen Memories", in J. Strachey, ed., *The Standard Edition of the Complete Psychological Works of Sigmund Freud*, trans. J. Strachey, Vol. III, London: Hogarth Press, pp. 299–322.

———, 1900, "The Interpretation of Dreams", in J. Strachey, ed., *The Standard Edition of the Complete Psychological Works of Sigmund Freud*, trans. J. Strachey, Vols. IV & V, London: Hogarth Press.

———, 1901, "The Psychopathology of Everyday Life", in J. Strachey, ed., *The Standard Edition of the Complete Psychological Works of Sigmund Freud,* trans. J. Strachey, Vol. VI, London: Hogarth Press.

———, 1905, "Three Essays on the Theory of Sexuality", in J. Strachey, ed., *The Standard Edition of the Complete Psychological Works of Sigmund Freud*, trans. J. Strachey, Vol. VII, London: Hogarth Press, pp. 125–144.

———, 1908, "Creative Writing and Day-Dreaming", in J. Strachey, ed., *The Standard Edition of the Complete Psychological Works of Sigmund Freud*, trans. J. Strachey, Vol. IX, London: Hogarth Press, pp. 141–154.

———, 1910, "The Antithetical Meaning of Primal Words", in J. Strachey, ed., *The Standard Edition of the Complete Psychological Works of Sigmund Freud*, trans. J. Strachey, Vol. XI, London: Hogarth Press, pp. 153–162.

———, 1912a, "The Handling of Dream-Interpretation in Psycho-Analysis", in J. Strachey, ed., *The Standard Edition of the Complete Psychological Works of Sigmund Freud,* trans. J. Strachey, Vol. XII, London: Hogarth Press, pp. 89–96.

———, 1912b, "Recommendations to Physicians Practicing Psycho-Analysis", in J. Strachey, ed., *The Standard Edition of the Complete Psychological Works of Sigmund Freud,* trans. J. Strachey, Vol. XII, London: Hogarth Press, pp. 109–121.

———, 1912c, "A Note on the Unconscious in Psycho-Analysis", in J. Strachey, ed., *The Standard Edition of the Complete Psychological Works of Sigmund Freud,* trans. J. Strachey, Vol. XII, London: Hogarth Press, pp. 255–266.

———, 1915, "Mourning and Melancholy", in J. Strachey, ed., *The Standard Edition of the Complete Psychological Works of Sigmund Freud,* trans. J. Strachey, Vol. XIV, London: Hogarth Press, pp. 237–258.

———, 1919, "The Uncanny", in J. Strachey, ed., *The Standard Edition of the Complete Psychological Works of Sigmund Freud,* trans. J. Strachey, Vol. XVII, London: Hogarth Press, pp. 217–256.

———, 1930, "Civilization and Its Discontents", in J. Strachey, ed., *The Standard Edition of the Complete Psychological Works of Sigmund Freud*, trans. J. Strachey, Vol. XXI, London: Hogarth Press, pp. 59–148.

———, 1937, "Constructions in Analysis", in J. Strachey, ed., *The Standard Edition of the Complete Psychological Works of Sigmund Freud*, trans. J. Strachey, Vol. XXIII, London: Hogarth Press, pp. 255–270.

———, 1954, *The Origins of Psycho-Analysis, Letters to Wilhelm Fliess, Drafts and Notes 1887–1902,* Marie Bonaparte, Anna Freud and Ernst Kris, eds., New York: Basic Books.

Freud, Sigmund and Andreas-Salomé, Lou, 1966, *Letters*, Pfeiffer, Ernst, ed., trans. Robson-Scott, William and Elaine, NY: Harcourt Brace Jovanovich, Inc., pp. 63–66.

Freud, Sigmund and Breuer, Joseph, 1893–1895, "Studies on Hysteria", in J. Strachey, ed., *The Standard Edition of the Complete Psychological Works of Sigmund Freud*, trans. J. Strachey, Vol. II, London: Hogarth Press.

Gadamer, Hans Georg, 2004, *Truth and Method*, 2nd Edition, New York: Continuum Press.

Gawsworth, John, 1969, "My Friend Lawrence Durrell", *Book Collecting & Library Monthly*, 15:80–81.

Gay, Peter, 1989, *Freud: A Life for our Time,* London: Papermac.

———, 1990, *Reading Freud*, New Haven: Yale University Press.

Gifford, James, 2003, "Durrell's the Revolt of Aphrodite: Nietzschean Influence", *Mosaic*, 36/2.

———, 2006, *The Unknown Is Constant*, Diss. University of Alberta, pp. 234–267.

———, 2007, "H. D.'s Hirslanden Notebooks & Durrell's Claudia: Occult Modernism Across the Curtain & in the Mirror." In *ANQ: A Quarterly Journal of Short Articles, Notes, & Reviews* 30/3:145–149.

———, 2008, "Vassanji's Toronto and Durrell's Alexandria: The View from Across or the View from Beside?" *The Journal of Commonwealth and Postcolonial Studies*, 15/2:28–43.

———, 2009, "Incest: A New Perspective", *Deus Loci*, 11:133–139.

Godshalk, William, 1967, "Some Sources of Lawrence Durrell's *Alexandria Quartet*", *Modern Fiction Studies*, 13:361–374.

Goldberg, Gerald, 1963, "The Search for the Artist in Some Recent British Fiction", *South Atlantic Quarterly*, 62:387–401.

Greenberg, Jay and Mitchell, Stephen, 1983, *Object Relations in Psychoanalytic Theory*, Harvard: Harvard University Press.

Griffiths, Gareth, 1978, *A Double Exile*, London: A. Marion Boyar Book.

Groddeck, Georg, 1961, *The Book of the It, Introduction by Lawrence Durrell,* London: Vision Press.

———, 1977, *The Meaning of Illness: Selected Psychoanalytic Writings Including His Correspondence with Sigmund Freud*, London: Hogarth Press and the Institute of Psycho-Analysis.

Gurr, Andrew, 1981, *Writers in Exile: The Identity of Home in Modern Literature*, Sussex, NJ: The Harvester Press and Humanities Press.

Haag, Michael, 2004, *Alexandria, City of Memory*, London: Yale University Press.

———, 2009, "To Alexandria with Eve Durrell", in *Deus Loci*, 11:3–6.

———, 2012a, *Lawrence Durrell: In an Irish Fairy's Armpit*, http://michaelhaag.blogspot.com/2012/11/lawrence-durrell-in-irish-fairys-armpit.html.

———, 2012b, "The *Alexandria Quartet* – from One Volume to Four", *Deus Loci*, 13:64–74.

———, 2017, *The Durrells of Corfu*, London: Profile Books.

Halim, Hala, 2006, "The City as Feminine Principle: The Feminization of Alexandria in Durrell's Clea", *Deus Loci*, 10.

———, 2013, *Alexandrian Cosmopolitanism: An Archive*, New York: Fordham University Press.

Hashem, Evine, 1991, "The City: The Unifying Element in Durrell's Justine", in Gindi Hoda, ed., *Images of Egypt in Twentieth Century Literature*, Cairo: University of Cairo, pp. 77–89.

Hirst, Anthony, 2004, "The Old Poet of the City: Cavafy in Darley's Alexandria", in *Lawrence Durrell and the Greek World*, London: Associated University Press, pp. 106–120.

Hodgkin, Joanna, 2013, *Amateurs in Eden: The Story of a Bohemian Marriage: Nancy and Lawrence Durrell*, London: Virago.

Hodes, Matthew, 1989, "Dreams Reconsidered", *Anthropology Today*, 5:6–8;

Hoffman, Frederick, 1945, *Freudianism and the Literary, Mind*, Baton Rouge: Louisiana State University Press.

Holland, Norman H., 1973, *Poems in Person*, New York: W. W. Norton & Company Inc.

Howarth, Herbert, 1972, "Durrell Snapped in a Library", *London Magazine*, 12:71–84.

Ingalls, Jeremy, 1994, "The Classics and New Poetry", *The Classical Journal*, 40:77–91.

Ingersoll, Earl G., 1998, *Lawrence Durrell: Conversations*, London: Associated University Press.

JanMohamed, Abdul R., 1985, "The Economy of Manichean Allegory: The Function of Racial Differences in Colonialist Literature", *Critical Inquiry*, 12:59–87.

Jasanoff, Maya, 2005, "Cosmopolitan a Tale from Ottoman Alexandria", *Common Knowledge*, 11/3:393–403.

Jones, Ernest, 1953–7, *The Life and Work of Sigmund Freud*, New York: Basic Books.

Jung, Carl, 1983, *Selected Writing*, ed. Anthony Storr, London: Fontana Press.

Kaczvinksy, Donald, 1993, "Classical and Medieval Sources for Lawrence Durrell", *Notes on Contemporary Literature*, 23:11–12.

Kaplan, Caren, 1996, *Questions of Travel, Postmodern Discourses of Displacement*, Durham: Duke University Press, pp. 125–129.

Kaufman, Barbara, 1995, "Training Tales in Family Therapy: Exploring *The Alexandria Quartet*", *Journal of Family and Marital Therapy*, 21:67–81.

Kersnowski, Frank, 2010, "The *Alexandria Quartet*: A Reconsideration", *Sewanee Review*, 118/3:381–392.

Kipling, Rudyard, 1993, *Kim*, Hertfordshire: Wordsworth Editions Limited.

Klein, Melanie, 1946, "Notes on Some Schizoid Mechanisms", in *The Collected Works of Melanie Klein*, Vol III. London: Hogarth Press and The Institute of Psycho-Analysis.

Knights, L. C., 1980, "Poetry and Things Hard for Thought", *International Review of Psychoanalysis*, 7:125–135.

Kohut, Heinz, 1957, "*Death in Venice* by Thomas Mann: A Story About the Disintegration of Artistic Sublimation", *Psychoanalysis Quarterly*, 26:206–228

Kristeva, Julia, 1987, *In the Beginning Was Love: Psychoanalysis and Faith*, trans. Arthur Goldhammer, New York: Columbia University Press.

———, 1991, *Strangers to Ourselves*, trans. L. S. Roudiez, New York: Columbia University Press.

Laplanche, Jean and Pontalis Jean, 1973, *The Language of Psychoanalysis*, New York: W. W. Norton & Company Inc.

Lejeune, Philippe, 1989, *On Autobiography*, ed. Paul John Eakin, Minneapolis: University of Minnesota Press.

Lipskar, Avidav, 2009, "Barriers: Liminal Thresholds in A. B. Yehoshua's Ethical Geography", *Democratic Culture*, 11:169–181.

Lorenz, Paul, 1995, "Who Is This Larry Durrell Character After All", *Thalia*, 15:24–31.

Lowenkron, David, 1976, "The Metanovel", *College English*, 38:345–355.

Lyttle, Andrew, 1966, *The Hero with Private Parts*, Baton Rouge: Louisiana State University Press.

Mackworth, Cecily, 1987, "Montparnasse and 18 Villa Seurat", *Twentieth Century Literature: A Scholarly and Critical Journal*, 33:274–279.

MacNiven, Ian S., 1988, ed., *The Durrell-Miller Letters*, 1935–1980, London: Faber & Faber.

———, 1998, *Lawrence Durrell: A Biography*, London: Faber & Faber.

———, 2005, "Lawrence Durrell", in *The Oxford Dictionary of National Biographies*, Oxford: Oxford University Press, pp. 324–230.

MacNiven, Ian S. and Moore, Harry T. eds. 1981, *Literary Lifelines: The Richard Aldington-Lawrence Durrell Correspondence*, New York: Viking Press.

Manzalaoui, Mahmoud, 1962, "Curate's Egg: An Alexandrian Opinion of Durrell's *Quartet*", *Etudes Anglaises*, 15:248–260.

Miller, Alice, 1987, *The Drama of Being a Child*, London: Virago Books.

Miller, Henry, 1934, *Tropic of Cancer*, New York: Grove Press.
———, 1945, *The Air-Conditioned Nightmare*, London: Granda Publishing.
———, 1949, *Sexus*, New York: Grove Press.
———, 1952, *The Books in My Life*, London: Viking Press.
Morcos, Mona, 1967, "Autobiographical Elements in *the Alexandrian Quartet*", *Modern Fiction Studies*, 13:343–359.
Moreno, Elie, 2011, "Once Upon in Egypt: Beaches and Bikinis from When Alexandria Was Club Med", *Foreign Policy*, April 27, pp. 36–48.
Morris, Jan, 2012, *"Introduction"*, in *the Alexandria Quartet*, London: Faber & Faber, pp. 4–9.
Morrison, Ray, 2007, *A Smile in his Mind's Eye: A Study of the Early Works of Lawrence Durrell*, Toronto: Toronto University Press.
Nägele, Rainer, 1978, *Reading After Freud*, New York: Columbia University Press.
Nietzsche, Friedrich, 1967a, *Ecce Homo*, trans. Walter Kaufmann, New York: Vintage Books.
———, 1967b, *On the Genealogy of Morals*, trans. Walter Kaufmann, New York: Vintage Books.
Nin, Anäis, 1967, *The Journals of Anäis Nin, Vol. 2: 1939–1944*, London: Quartet Books.
———, 1976, *The Journals of Anäis Nin, Vol. 6: 1955–1966*, London: Quartet Books.
———, 1980, *The Journals of Anäis Nin, Vol. 7: 1966–1974*, London: Quartet Books.
Ogden, Thomas, 1997, "Some Thoughts on the Use of Language in Psychoanalysis", *Psychoanalytic Dialogues*, 7:1–21.
———, 2000, "Borges and the Art of Mourning", *Psychoanalytic Dialogues*, 10:65–88.
Ogden, Thomas and Benjamin Ogden, 2013, *The Analyst's Ear and the Critic's Ear*, London & New York: Routledge.
Orwell, George, 1957, *Inside the Whale*, London: Penguin Books.
Parker, Kim, 1993, "Home Is Where the Heart Lies", *Transition*, 59:65–77.
Pedaya, Haviva, 2011, *Walking Through Trauma: Rituals of Movement in Jewish Myth, Mysticism, and History (Hebrew)*, Tel Aviv: Resling Publishing Ltd.
Perlès, Alfred, 1961, *My Friend Lawrence Durrell*, Northwood: Scorpion Press.
Pine, Richard, 2005, *Lawrence Durrell: The Mindscape*, Corfu: The Durrell School of Corfu.
———, 2018, "Lawrence Durrell's Minor Mythologies" in *his Minor Mythologies as Popular Literature*, Cambridge: Cambridge Scholars Publishing.
Plutarch, 1958, *The Lives of the Noble Grecians and Romans*, New York: Bennet and Klopfer.
Porter, Roger, 2001, "Autobiography, Exile, Home: The Egyptian Memoirs of Gini Alhadef, Andre Aciman and Edward Said", *Biography*, 24:302–313.
Quinodoz, Jean-Michel, 2005, *Reading Freud*, London & New York: Routledge.
Rank, Otto, 1932, *The Myth of the Birth of the Hero*, trans. Gregory C. Richter and E. James Lieberman, New York: Vintage Books.
Robson, Barbara, 1991, "The Darker Side of Durrell", *The Sunday Telegraph*, May 26, pp. 23–26.
Roth, Merav, 2019, *Reading the Reader – A Psychoanalytic Perspective on Literature*, London and New York: Routledge.
Rushdie, Salman, 1991, *Imaginary Homelands: Essays and Criticism 1981–1991*, London: Penguin Books.
Sagi, Avi, 2009, *The Human Voyage to Meaning: A Philosophical-Hermeneutical Study of Literary Works [Hebrew]*, Ramat-Gan: Bar-Ilan University Press.
Sandler, Joseph, Dare Christopher and Hope Alex, 1992, *The Patient and the Analyst*, London: Karnac Books.
Schleiermacher, Friedrich, 1977, *Two Academy Addresses of 1829: On the Concept of Hermeneutics, Hermeneutics: The Handwritten Manuscripts*, ed. Heinz Kimmerle and trans. Duke James and Forstman Jack, Missoula: Scholar Press.

Seidel, Michael, 1986, *Exile and the Narrative Imagination*, New Haven and London: Yale University Press.

Simpson, John, ed. 1995, *The Oxford Book of Exile*, Oxford and New York: Oxford University Press.

Sligh, Charles L., 1998, "Reading the Divergent Weave: A Note and Some Speculations on Durrell and Cortázar", *Deus Loci*, 6:118–132.

Spence, Donald, 1982, *Narrative Truth and Historical Truth*, New York: W. W. Norton & Company Inc.

———, 2003, "Listening for Rhetorical Truth", *Psychoanalytical Quarterly*, 83:875–903.

Spero, Moshe Halevi, 2010, "The Transformations in the 'Mental Apparatus of Dreaming' as Depicted in the Biblical Story of Joseph (Genesis 40–43)", in L. Aron and Libby Henik, eds., *Contemporary Psychoanalysis and Judaism*, New York: Academic Studies Press, p. 186.

———, 2018, "The Unique Contribution of Hebrew to the Conceptualization of the Psychodynamic Psychotherapy", in Rony Alfandary, ed., *Seeking Psychic Space: Fundamentals of Psychodynamic Social Work, (Hebrew)*, Jerusalem: Carmel Publishers, pp. 291–322.

Steiner, George, 1961, *The Death of Tragedy*, London: Faber & Faber.

———, 1967, *Language and Silence*, London: Faber & Faber.

———, 1978, *On Difficulty*, Oxford: Oxford University Press.

———, 1989, *Real Presences*, London: Faber & Faber.

Storr, Anthony, 1988, *Solitude*, New York: Ballantine Books.

Swift, Jonathan, 1997, *Gulliver's Travels*, Herts: Wordsworth Editions Ltd.

Thompson, Edward, 1989, "The Writer in Exile, the Good Years", *Slavic and East European Journal*, 33/4:124–156.

Turner, Victor, 1969, *The Ritual Process*, New Brunswick and London: Aldine transaction.

Unterecker, John, 1964, *Lawrence Durrell*, New York and London: Columbia University Press.

Walsh, W. H., 1958, "Plain and Significant Narrative," *History Journal of Philosophy*, 55:479–484.

Weigel, John A., 1965, *Lawrence Durrell*, New York: Twayne Publishers Inc.

Whitman, Aldan, 1970, "Durrell in Despair of Future of Man", *New York Times*, March 20.

Wickes, George, 1963, *Lawrence Durrell & Henry Miller: A Private Correspondence: Letters of Lawrence Durrell and Henry Miller 1935–1959*, London: E. P. Dutton & Co., Inc.

Williams, Gwyn, 1987, "Durrell in Egypt", *Twentieth Century Literature: A Scholarly and Critical Journal*, 33:298–302.

Winnicott, D. W., 1960, *The Maturational Processes and the Facilitating Environment*, London: Karnac Books.

———, 1971, *Therapeutic Consultations in Child Psychiatry*, London: Karnac Books.

Young, Kenneth, 1959, "A Dialogue with Durrell", *Encounter*, 1/6:62.

Zahaln, Anne, 1986, "The Destruction of the Imperial Self in Lawrence Durrell's The *Alexandria Quartet*", *Perspectives on Contemporary Literature*, 12:3–16.

Ziffer, Benny, 2017, "Why was I so happy to see Alfandary's Exile and Return" (Hebrew), in *Haaretz*, January 11th, https://www.haaretz.co.il/literature/study/1.3230353

INDEX

Agon 123, 124, 136n64
Alexandre-Garner, Corinne 11n17, 105n6; *Etude sur l'amour, la femme et l'ecriture* viii
Adam, Peter 88, 105n7
Abel, Carl 58, 72n10
Acker, Kathy 9–10
Acoustic illusion 94
Africa 29, 86
Alexander the Great 89
Alexandre-Garner, Corinne 11n17, 105n6; *Etude sur l'amour, la femme et l'ecriture* viii
Alexandria, the city 28, 102; Mother-City 93–96
Alexandria Quartet, The vi, 4–5, 10n1, 13–14, 54nn7–8
Alfandary, Rony 34n56, 72n11
Alter-ego 14, 32n8, 48
Amaril (A character in the *Quartet*) 102
Andreas-Salomé, Lou 101
Anglo-Indian 1, 30, 72n10, 84, 112, 114, 119, 120, 121
Anglo-Saxon 4, 5, 69, 90
Angry Young Men 9
Antony, Mark 51–52, 100
Apathy 90
Appelfeld, Aharon: *Poland, A Green Land* 15
Arab 86
Arcturus 95–96, 109n85
Armstrong, James 109n94
Art/Artist 5, 7, 17, 24, 31, 79, 80, 82, 83, 84, 128
Arnauti, Jacob (A character in the *Quartet*) 48, 61, 100
Auden, W.H. 21
Author/Writer 33, 82; authentic voice 9; authority 44; author, narrator, writer, 32n2; the author, *the Heraldic Universe* and loneliness 79–87; biographical element 14, 15, 16–17, 18; coming of age of the author 125–129; consciousness 40, 46, 94, 98, 112; exiled 26, 28–32, 96, 105; fragmented nature 30–32; imagination 21, 24, 25, 39, 71, 78, 85; inner world 85; intentions 39, 41, 43; ironic intention 38; isolation 3–4; loss 27; maturational process 37; motivation 22, 70; personal experiences 111; "real" 127; reflective process 24, 25, 39, 41, 75, 138, 139, 140; repressed childhood 16; unconscious 21, 22, 24, 94
Avignon Quintet, The viii, xi, 41, 43
Azoulay, Ariella 28

Bachelard, Gaston 76, 95, 139
Bakhtin, Michail 16–17
Balthazar (character in the *Quartet*) 19, 48, 51, 52–53, 61–62, 63, 86, 96, 100, 101, 103, 121–122, 130
Balthazar (Second volume of the *Quartet*) 11n4, 13, 14, 37, 42, 43, 45, 52, 61, 63, 71, 94, 120
Barchilon, Jose 21
Baroque 8

Barthes, Roland 15; *Death of the Author* 39; *Mythologies* 27, 85
Bauman, Zygmunt 11n15, 30, 35n80
Begnal, Michael H. 8
Belfer, Ella 29, 69
Beckett, Samuel 26
Belgrade 79
Ben-Gurion, David 2
Benjamin, Walter: *The Work of Art in the Age of Mechanical Reproduction* 28
Bergson, Henri 43
Bhabha, Homi 27, 87
Bildungsroman 38, 49
Biographical/Fictional elements in literature 14–18
Bion, Wilfred R. 58, 59
Birthplace 1, 22, 23–24, 26, 69, 112, 114
Bisexuality 97–98, 100–101, 109n93
Bitter Lemons 12n40, 118, 135n42
Black Book, The viii, x, 4, 5, 6, 30, 35n82, 41, 104, 109n94, 112, 126, 127, 128, 136n63
Blake, William 21
Bloom, Harold 3–4, 14, 44, 55n31; *The Anxiety of Influence* 127
Boarding school/School: 131, 137n80; England 3, 112, 118, 120, 121, 122, 127, 128; Jesuit ix, 120; St. Edmund's ix; St. Joseph's ix, 118, 119
Bollas, Christopher 54n23, 58, 72n7, 106n11; *Forces of Destiny* 76–77
Bode, Carl 78
Bonaparte, Marie 15, 32n11, 109n93
Bonaparte, Napoleon 32n11
Borges, Jorge Luis 21
Boysson, Ghislaine de (wife) 131
Botting, Douglas 113, 116
Bowker, Gordon 93, 113, 115, 117, 119, 121, 129, 133
Brassaï 6
Breuer, Joseph: *Studies on Hysteria* 109n93
Breton, André 6
Brewster, Chamberlin 11n21
Brink, André 9
Brink, Andrew 22
British intelligence/Foreign Office/Council/Administration 19, 49, 52, 69, 89, 93, 129
Bruno, Giordano 59, 72n18
Buddhist/Taoist/Zen 7, 81, 114
Burgess, Anthony 9

Cairo 90
Callisto (Ursa Major) 109n85
Cavafy, Constantine P.: *The God Abandons Antony* 51–52, 55n42, 55n44
Camus, Albert 21, 33n35
Capodistria (character in the *Quartet*) 19, 101
Casement, Patrick 133, 137n96
Censorship 6, 97–98, 100, 109n94
Chania 887
Chasseguet-Smirgel, Janine 104, 110n120
Christian 88, 110n116
City, The 76
Clawson, James M. 9, 12n46
Clea (character in the *Quartet*) 7, 19, 36, 49, 82, 99, 100
Clea (Third volume of the *Quartet*) 38, 39, 42, 43–44, 49, 54n8, 57, 63, 100, 102, 134n4, 136n65, 136n67, 136n76
Cleyet, George 11n20
Cleopatra 51, 100, 103, 110n116
Clinical 20, 25, 34n56, 101, 137n96
Cohen, Eve Yvette (wife) 2, 89, 121, 129
Colas, Santiago 55n30
Colonialism 1, 69, 84, 85, 86, 87, 93, 114, 117; post 86
Condensation 15, 20, 57
Conflict 24, 45, 53, 66, 69, 94, 95, 98
Conrad, Joseph 26
Consciousness 3, 8, 15, 19, 24, 32, 46, 66, 70, 75, 78, 79, 87, 94, 102, 103, 104, 105, 112, 120, 140; altered- 65; author 40; deep 98; dreamer 60; individual 40; loss of 64; state of 64; stream-of 36
Contemporary context 1–10; cultural contexts 3–5; influence 8–10; literary beginnings 5–6; politics and style 6–8
Continuum 31; associative 44; chronological 38; cognitive 59; conscious 46; emotional 59; idiosyncratic 36; linear 37; narrative 37; plot 41; reflective 46; word 41, 43, 79
Coptic/Copts 18, 19, 49, 67, 68, 69, 86, 88, 92, 131
Corfu viii, x, 5, 10, 11n3, 11n21, 26, 81, 116, 122, 123, 125, 128, 134n14
Correspondence: angry letters from readers 77; Durrell 18, 106n16, 113, 134n17; Durrell from 1930s 6, 28; Durrell from 1940s 75–76, 77, 89, 93; Durrell in Alexandria 75, 87–93; Durrell in Corfu 125–126; Durrell in the *Quartet* 46, 89, 93; Durrell 1941–1945 87–93; Durrell omitting dates 54n10; Durrell's painful experiences 90; Durrell with Allan G. Thomas 136n68; Durrell with Miller 7, 23, 34n44. 106n23, 113, 126, 127, 131; Durrell while writing *Justine* 43; Fliess 97, 109n93; Freud 32n11, 97, 109n93; love 130; Pursewarden 49; Sappho 132, 133

Cortázar, Julio 9, 44, 55n31
Creativity 7, 14, 21, 24, 31, 37, 45, 70, 75, 80, 82, 129
Crete 87, 108n63
Cyprus 26, 79, 87, 125, 129, 132, 137nn79–80

Dawson, Carl 12n31
Darjeeling 117, 118
Dark Labyrinth, The viii, x
Darley, L. G. (A character in the *Quartet*) 5, 7, 13, 17, 18, 19, 22, 23, 24, 25, 30, 33n21, 36, 38, 39, 46, 48–53, 55n29, 56, 57, 60–63, 67, 68, 71, 74, 83, 84, 93, 94, 96, 98, 99, 100, 101, 102, 103, 105, 115
Darwish, Mahmoud 31
Defence mechanisms 42, 57, 63, 98
De Sade, Marquis: *Justine, or The Misfortunes of Virtue* 62, 73n21, 104, 110n122
Destiny 38, 61, 71, 75, 76, 84–85, 95, 96, 99, 123
Dearborn, Mary V. 134n5
Deep, Marquis 86, 107n48
Derrida, Jacques 26–27, 29, 35n61, 35n77
Diboll, Mike 55n35
Death 27, 29, 46, 53, 89, 90, 102; Alexandrian 90, 92, 96, 100; Antony, Mark 51; Durrell, Lawrence George 15, 79, 82, 88, 108n64, 112, 129, 131, 133–134; Durrell, Claude (Durrell's third wife) 9, 81, 130, 131, 132, 133; Durrell, Lawrence Samuel (Durrell's father), 110n114, 120–122, 128; Durrell, Margery (Durrell's sister) 115, 117; English 8, 104, 122–125, 128; Freud 23; Leila's husband 110n14; Mann, Thomas' mother 22; Miller 106n23, 127, 128; renunciation 44; Shakespeare, Hamnet 18; Steiner 74; writers 1
Destruction of history 44
Deus Loci 10
Diary/Diaries 46; Death Gregory 123; Durrell, Lawrence George 111; Durrell, Sappho 9, 115, 131–132, 133; Justine 48; Nessim Hosnani 48; Nin, Anaïs 111; Pursewarden 39, 49
Dibdin, Michael 120
Dickinson, Emily 21
Disease 84, 90, 99, 102, 115, 135n30; *see also* illness; sickness
Dixie, George 114
Double/Doppelgänger 2, 32n8, 49
Dreams and dreaming 56–71; aspiration for truth 70–71; dream as a structure 59–64; Mountolive 64–65; Nessim 66–70
Drive 25, 26, 53, 64, 70, 71, 122; sexual 73n27
Durrell, Lawrence George
  The Alexandria Quartet vi, 4–5, 10n1, 13–14, 54nn7–8; Alexandria as the mother-city 93–96; "author," "narrator," "writer," 32n2; belonging and exile 26–28, 30; biographical and fictional elements 14, 16–18; bisexuality 100–101; dreams and dreaming 56, 57, 59, 60, 62, 63, 64, 71; healing power of writing 56; historical truth 71; identity 83; Marxism 7; Mountolive's dream 64–65; narrative labyrinth 36; narrative time and narrative voices 37–40; narrator 31; narrator as critical commentator 52–53; narrator as wounded hero 50–52; Nessim's dream 66–70; 1941–1945 correspondence 87–93; Nobel nominations 2; plot 46–47, 98; Oriental Other 85; prefatory notes and narrative voices 40–44; psychoanalysis interpretation vii, viii, 3, 13, 22–26; sexuality 5, 6, 55n40, 97–99, 100–101, 104; structure 42, 44–46; theory of relativity 43–44; therapeutic use 34n40; three layers of plot 46–47; topographic return to Alexandria 76–79; translations 10, 11n4, 55n31; voices of the narrative 47–50; wish 104–105; writing x, 32, 129–131; *see also* Amaril; *Balthazar*; *Clea*; Darley; Dreams and dreaming; Homeland; *Justine*; *Mountolive*; Narrative voices; Orient/Oriental; Plot; Pursewarden
  Ancestry 11n5, 32, 69, 120, 122
  Avignon Quintet, The viii, xi, 41, 43
  Balthazar (Second volume of the *Quartet*) 11n4, 13, 14, 37, 42, 43, 45, 52, 61, 63, 71, 94, 120
  Belonging and exile 26–28
  Birth ix, 1, 10, 22, 23, 25, 26, 69, 112, 114–115, 116, 134n11; Greece as second place 88; literary rebirth 126
  Bitter Lemons 12n40, 118, 135n42
  Black Book, The viii, x, 4, 5, 6, 30, 35n82, 41, 104, 109n94, 112, 126, 127, 128, 136n63
  Book of the Dead, The 92, 108n63
  Booster\Delta 12n24
  Censorship 6, 97–98, 100, 109n94
  Childhood *Kim* years 113–115

Clea (Third volume of the *Quartet*) 38, 39, 42, 43–44, 49, 54n8, 57, 63, 100, 102, 134n4, 136n65, 136n67, 136n76
Dark Labyrinth, The viii, x
Death 15, 79, 82, 88, 108n64, 112, 129, 131, 133–134
Egypt 2, 19, 26, 38, 45, 49, 51, 52, 67, 79, 86, 88, 89, 90, 106n12, 129; British Protectorate 73n30; Coptic 68, 69, 131; exile 125; War 93; *see also Lavon Affair*
England 3, 26, 69, 112, 114, 118, 119, 120–121, 122, 124, 125, 127
English Death 7, 104; *The Black Book* 122–125
Exile 28–30; belonging 26–28; Egypt 125; England 3, 26, 69, 112, 114, 118, 119, 120–121, 122, 124, 125, 127; leaving 118–120
Daughters *see* Durrell, Penelope; Durrell, Sappho
French citizenship 11n6
Greece 11n3, 18, 19, 26, 27, 57, 60, 61, 69, 78, 87, 88, 90, 91, 92, 93, 96, 103, 106n19, 123, 124, 128, 131; coming of age of the author 125–129
Happy decade and lost children 131–133
Heraldic Universe, the 7, 14, 79–87, 96, 107n26, 127, 133, 140
Influence 8–10
Judith viii, 2, 10
Justine (First volume of the *Quartet*) x, 11n16, 11n19, 13, 23, 24, 32n1, 32n5, 33n23, 34n39, 34n44, 34n47, 34n49, 36, 41, 49, 51, 53, 53n1, 54n6, 54n11, 55n36, 55n38, 55n41, 72n2, 73n20, 73n28, 105n2, 107n31, 107n38, 107n41, 107n49, 108n77, 108n79, 108n84, 109n84, 109n97, 110n102, 110n106, 134n10; Alexandria as the mother-city 93, 95, 96, 97, 98, 99, 100, 103; characters as invention 42; city is real 42; consciousness 112; diaries 48; dreams and dreaming 60–61, 63, 66, 68; exile 18; fate of man 100; fiftieth anniversary 106n12; length of time of writing 42–43, 129, 130; mother-city 78; plot 45, 52; sexuality 100, 104; sickness 84, 115; solitude 83; splendours of ocean 14; translation 11n4; travelling 118; wish 56
Justine 2 61
Marriages (Nancy, Eve, Claude, Ghislaine) 75, 78, 89, 93, 102, 108n64, 114, 129; *see also* Boysson, Ghislaine de; Cohen, Eve Yvette; Myers, Nancy Isabel; Vincendon, Claude-Marie/Claude
Mediterranean Shore, The viii
Modern love 5, 13, 50, 68, 70
Mother-City 74–105; Alexandria as 93–96; author, *the Heraldic Universe* and loneliness 79–87; Durrell, Freud, Fliess and bisexuality 96–100; Durrell, Groddeck, sexuality and death 100–102; the return 102–105; topographic return to Alexandria 76–79
Mountolive (Third volume of the *Quartet*) x, 12n27, 28, 32n4, 34n41, 35n66, 35n81, 42, 49, 55n29, 73n25, 73n31, 73n33, 73n35, 102, 135n46, 136n54, 136n58; dream 62, 63–66, 68, 71
Nunquam viii, xi, 10, 36
Panic Spring x, 136n63
Parents *see* Durrell, Louisa; Durrell, Lawrence Samuel
Paris viii, 127, 128; 1937 x, 6, 81, 130; 1938: publication of *The Black Book* x, 35n82
Personal Landscape x
Placebo, The viii, 10
Politics and style 6–8
Prospero's Cell x
Pudding Island 5, 7
Spirit of Place 106n16, 108n66, 108n71, 135n23, 136n68, 136n77, 137n99
Smile in the Mind's Eye, A 54n9, 81, 105n4, 107n25, 107n28, 112, 134n9, 135n25
Style 6–8
Tunc vii, viii, xi, 10, 32n13, 36
Durrell, Lawrence Samuel (father) 113, 117, 120, 121, 122, 127, 135n38
Durrell, Leslie Stewart (brother) ix, 117, 119
Durrell, Gerald (brother) 38, 113, 132; *My Family and Other Animals* 2, 11n3, 116, 135n35
Durrell, Louisa (mother) 113, 114, 115–118, 119
Durrell, Margaret "Margo" (sister) ix, 116, 117, 119, 132
Durrell, Margery (sister) ix, 115, 117, 119, 132
Durrell, Penelope (daughter) x, 89, 128, 129
Durrell, Samuel Lawrence 113–114
Durrell, Sappho (daughter) x, 12n48, 89, 113, 114, 116, 119, 130, 134n18, 135n26, 135n31, 136n59, 136n55, 137n92; diaries 9, 115, 121, 131–132, 133

Durrell School of Corfu/Durrell Library of Corfu 134n14
Durrells, The (TV series) 10

Eagleton, Terry 9, 12n46
Eskin, Stanley 53n2
Eden 28, 69, 76, 102, 139
Ego, the 52, 53, 81
Egypt 2, 19, 26, 38, 45, 49, 51, 52, 67, 79, 86, 88, 89, 90, 106n12, 129; British Protectorate 73n30; Coptic 68, 69, 131; exile 125; War 93; *see also Lavon Affair*
Einstein, Albert 39, 43, 44, 139
Eliot, T.S. 4, 6, 8, 54n11, 109n94, 110n119, 122
Elizabethan 6, 7, 8, 22, 129
Elusive memory 46
England/English 1, 104; Durrell attends boarding school 3, 26, 69, 112, 114, 118, 119, 120–121, 122, 124, 125, 127; Durrell leaves viii, 5, 32, 124, 125, 128; The Durrells move from 116; Louisa (mother) and siblings return 128; 1924: Louisa visits ix; 1925: The Durrells visit Lawrence ix; 1926: Lawrence Samuel visits ix; 1930s sexual oppression 110n119; 1964: Louisa dies in x
English death 7, 104, 122–125, 128
Europe 5, 23, 47, 88, 93, 114, 120; refugees 86, 89
Exile 118–120; belonging 26–28; England 3, 26, 69, 112, 114, 118, 119, 120–121, 122, 124, 125, 127
Exiled writer 26, 28–32, 96, 105; fragmented nature 30–32

Faber & Faber 4, 35n82, 109n94, 122, 131, 136n63
Father: death 120–122; figure 3, 110n109, 121, 127, 119
Felman, Shoshana: 19, 33n26; *Testimony* 17, 33n18, 132, 137n89
Feminism 25
Festa-McCormick, Diana 86, 107n50
Finch, Peter 2
Fliess, Wilhelm 97, 100, 109n93
Forde, Barry (Claude-Marie Vincendon's son) 129
Forde, Dianna (Claude-Marie Vincendon's daughter) 129
Forde, Claude-Marie (Vincendon) (third Wife) 43; death 9, 81, 130, 131, 132, 133
Forde, Tim 129
Forster, E. M. 77
Foreign Office 93, 129
Franklin, Steve 38–39, 54n17
Fraser, G. S. 34n43
Freud, Sigmund i, viii, 15, 32n6, 33n22, 35n60, 54n7, 55n32, 72n6, 72n9, 73n24, 115; bisexuality 98, 100; censorship 97, 98; *Civilization and Its Discontents* 14; *Constructions in Analysis* 70, 73n36; *Creative Writers and Day-Dreaming* 24, 34n52, 55n34; depression 54n23; dominance of unconscious 44; dreams 23, 57, 58, 60, 63, 64, 66, 67; escape from Nazi occupied Vienna 32n11; father figure 3, 110n109; Fliess relationship 97109n93; *A Fragment of an Analysis of a Case of Hysteria* 97; Groddeck relationship 110n109; *The Handling of Dream-Interpretation in Psycho-Analysis* 34n44; *Heimlich* 1; I (*ich*) 101, 110n111; infantile sexuality 23; interpretation of dreams 45, 60, 66; *The Interpretation of Dreams* 58; misreading 23; *Mourning and Melancholy* 54n23, 106n9; *nachträglich* 27; naming protagonist 17–18; Nietzsche 83; ocean metaphor 14; *The Origins of Psychoanalysis* 34n44, 109n91; psychoanalysis 19–20, 21, 23, 24, 48; *Recommendations to Physicians Practising Psycho-Analysis* 34n55; religion 14; return of the repressed 94; Rolland correspondence 14; sexuality 23, 25, 45, 73n27, 97; The Shadow of the Object 54n23; similarity between Hamlet and Hamnet 18; slips of the tongue 23; *Studies of Hysteria* 97, 109n93; superego 32n8; topographical models of the mind 10, 44–45; truth 70;; unconscious 44, 45, 57, 83, 96, 140; das *unheimliche* (*The Uncanny*) 1, 2, 14, 22, 26, 27, 30, 32n8, 42, 45, 46, 56, 58, 65, 67, 69, 71, 90, 93, 94, 95, 103, 114, 120, 123, 124, 134, 138, 139
Friedman, Alan Warren: *Art for Love's Sake* viii

Gadamer, Hans-Georg 16, 33n15, 39, 40, 54n19, 54n26
Gascoyne, David 6
Gawsworth, John 7–8, 12n33
Gay, Peter 33n28, 109n93
German Luftwaffe 87
Gide, André: *The Counterfeiters* 39
Gifford, James 107n26, 107n34, 109n95, 113, 132, 137n94
Godshalk, William 12n30

Goldberg, Gerald 38, 54n14
Greenberg, Jay 34n58, 106n9
Gregory, Death (character in *The Black Book*) 123, 124
Gide, André: *The Counterfeiters* 39
Goethe, Johann Wolfgang von 20
Greece/Greek 89, 110n116; Ancient 7, 96; Durrell 11n3, 18, 19, 26, 27, 57, 60, 61, 69, 78, 87, 88, 90, 91, 92, 93, 96, 103, 106n19, 123, 124, 128, 131; Durrell coming of age 125–129; mythology 96; *see also Agon*; Corfu
Griffiths, Gareth 29, 35n76
Groddeck, Georg 3, 23, 48, 100, 110nn108–109, 110n113; bisexuality 101; *The Book of It* 100; "The Ego and the Id" 110n109; das *ich* 110n111; *The Meaning of Illness* 110n103, 110n105, 110n110, 110n112
Grotstein, James 58
Gulliver 64, 65
Gurr, Andrew 28, 35n69

Haag, Michael 11n3, 11n5, 40, 42, 54n11, 54n25, 55n28, 68, 108n60, 113, 130, 137n85; "To Alexandria with Eve Durrell" 108n64
Haggard, Rider 117; *King Solomon's Mines* 135n41
Hashem, Evine 78, 106n17
Halim, Hala 106n12
Hamlet 18; *see also* Shakespeare, William: *Hamlet*
Hebrew 1, 11n4, 11n10, 32n9, 58, 73n29
Hebrew University 109n93
Hemingway, Ernest 8
Henty, George: *The Lion of St. Mark* 117
Hera 109n85
Hermeneutic 16, 39, 138
Hero 102; anti- 123; wounded 50–52
Hirst, Anthony 55n45
Hodgkin, Joanna 11n21
Hodes, Matthew 73n19
Hoffman, Frederick 73n19
Hoffman E.T.A. 1
Hogarth, Paul: *The Mediterranean Shore* viii
Holland, Norman H. 16, 33n16
Holocaust 2
Homeland i, 26, 28, 31, 42, 67, 88, 90, 95, 104, 127, 134; ancestral 69, 122; British 120, 125; cultural 1, 124; homemade 81; imaginary 23, 24, 29, 30, 32, 47, 63, 75, 82, 93, 138, 139; Jewish 3; language 26; loathsome 124; lost 31, 76, 81, 105, 133; Nietzsche 83; oppressive 70; The Other 27; primeval 10, 22, 74, 105, 117; *unheimliche* 67, 139; *see also Heraldic Universe*
Howarth, Herbert 38, 54n16, 77, 106n13
Hysterical identification 17

Isaac, Binding of 120
Identity 2, 5, 13, 71, 75, 83, 95, 98, 100, 114, 119, 120, 131, 140; artist 80; collective 29, 69; conspirators 68; destabilised 31; narrative voice 66; narrator 31, 50; non-cohesive 48; plural 47; subjective 32; undisclosed 49; writer 31, 138
Imaginary homeland 23, 24, 30, 32, 47, 63, 75, 82, 138, 139
Imperialism 9, 85, 86, 88, 106n12, 114, 118
Incest, 104, 108n63, 132
India: colonial 86; Durrell leaves ix, 26, 75, 120, 121; Durrell's birthplace ix, 1, 3, 14, 22, 23–24, 28, 32, 32n2, 69, 112, 113; Durrell's childhood 69, 86, 87, 88, 113–114, 130, 135n30, 136n53; exile 93, 112, 118, 119, 121, 122, 129; homeland 88, 104, 122; imperialism 114; independence 115; infant mortality 115; Jalandhar ix; Lawrence Samuel dies ix; Louisa and children leave ix; Louisa visits England and returns ix; Orwell 31; parents and sister return ix
Ingalls, Jeremy 12n35
Ingersoll, Earl G. 12n32, 55n39, 108n57, 134n8
Instincts 77, 80, 84, 94
Interlinear, the 48, 53, 61
International Lawrence Durrell Society 10, 113
Interpretation 1, 9, 10, 15, 17, 36, 37, 39, 44, 50, 54n7, 79, 87, 101, 134n11, 138; clinical 20; dreams 20, 45, 56, 57, 58, 61, 62, 63, 66; letters 76, 87–93; multi-dimensional 52; prose 76; psychoanalytic 16, 22–26; silence 24; textual 14, 20, 22, 57, 75
Irish 7, 11n5, 33n21, 116, 129
Ishiguro, Kazuo 9
Israel vi, 1, 2, 4, 10, 15, 27, 59, 68, 135n45, 137n82, 137n86
Id 37, 45
Illness 110n108; mental 98; *see also* disease; sickness
It (Groddeck's term) viii, 100–101, 110n109, 110n113

James, Duke 33n14
James, Henry 78
JanMohamed, Abdul R. 87, 107n53

Jasanoff, Maya 108n59
Jerusalem 89, 90, 109n93
Jews/Jewish 2–3, 7, 18, 19, 29, 86, 89, 129; Alexandria 68; Egyptian 137n86; independence 68; Palestine 49, 69; underground 49, 68, 88
Jewish underground 2, 19, 49, 68, 88
Joyce, James 4, 28
Jones, Ernest 107n35, 109n93
Jalandhar (Jullundur) 114
Judith viii, 2, 10
Jung, Carl viii, 3, 66–67, 73n27
Justine (A character in the *Quartet*) 2, 18, 19, 23, 25, 36, 49, 51, 53, 89; diaries 48; dreams and dreaming 67, 68; prototype of all women 99; "truth" 52
Justine (First volume of the *Quartet*) x, 11n16, 11n19, 13, 23, 24, 32n1, 32n5, 33n23, 34n39, 34n44, 34n47, 34n49, 36, 41, 49, 51, 53, 53n1, 54n6, 54n11, 55n36, 55n38, 55n41, 72n2, 73n20, 73n28, 105n2, 107n31, 107n38, 107n41, 107n49, 108n77, 108n79, 108n84, 109n84, 109n97, 110n102, 110n106, 134n10

Kabballah 19, 52
Kaczvinksy, Donald 12n29
Kaplan, Caren 11n18
Kaufman, Barbara 34n40, 107n36, 107nn39–40, 107n42, 108n78
Kersnowski, Frank 40, 54n22
Keats, John (A character in the *Quartet*) 3
Kestsman, Françoise (Durrell's last female partner) 131, 133
Kipling, Rudyard: *Kim* 114, 117, 135n22, 135n30
Klein, Melanie 11n10, 25, 34n58, 107n44
Knights, L. C. 21, 33n31
Kohut, Heinz 22, 33n36
Kristeva, Julia vii, 18, 31, 33n24, 35n84, 55n37, 95, 108n83, 111, 134n1
Kurseong 117

Language 4, 7, 8, 15, 19, 22, 23, 25, 26, 77, 87, 94, 97, 137n79, 138; ancient 58; Anglo-Indian 72n10; dreams 56, 57, 71; exiled writer 28; fictional and deliberate 14; foreign 26, 29; homeland 26; inspiring 10; nature 58, 140; obscene 10; realm 71; rich 14, 16, 88, 123; Semitic 72n10; sexuality 98; writer's 31
Laplanche, Jean: *The Language of Psychoanalysis* 54n7
Latent 20, 21, 23, 57, 63, 64, 67, 68, 69
Latin 7
Latin American Boom 44
Lawrence, D. H. 8, 10, 111, 134n4
Laub, Dori: *Testimony* 17, 33n18, 132, 137n89
Lavon Affair 130, 137n86
Leila (A character in the *Quartet*) 19, 22, 102, 110n114
Lessing, Doris: *The Golden Notebook* 39
Lejeune, Philippe 17, 33n19
Lipskar, Avidav 4, 11n9
Letters *see* Correspondence
Lieberman, E. James 135n27
Lilliput, land of 65
Liminal: city 74; experience 75, 84; phenomenon 98; process 98, 122; quality 97; space 28, 76, 88, 93, 103, 105, 115, 138, 140; stage 10; state 102
Lisa (A character in the *Quartet*) 19, 55n40
Literature, biographical/fictional elements 14–18; psychoanalysis 19–22
London viii, 11n21, 78, 85; Eve Durrell 108n64; exile 23; Freud 32n11; Hotel Regina 123; moved away 11n21; 1924: schooling ix; 1929: Lawrence spends more time ix; 1931: moves and publishes his first collection of poetry ix; 1935: marries Nancy x; Mountolive 28; periodical return 28; Sappho psychoanalysis 133; Southwark ix; 2012: Centenary conference 12n51; *see also* Faber & Faber
Lorenz, Paul 39, 54n20
Loneliness 26, 61, 80, 82, 114, 119, 133
Loren, Sophia 2
Lorenz, Paul 39, 54n20
Lowenkron, David 39, 54n21
Lucifer, Lawrence (character in *The Black Book*) 123, 124, 125
Lycaon 109n85
Lyttle, Andrew 55n27

Mackworth, Cecily 12n25
MacNiven, Ian S. 11n12, 12n22, 12n24, 12n26, 12n50, 34n45, 72n18, 73n29, 79, 86, 106n19, 106n21, 106n23, 107n24, 107n29, 107n47, 107n55, 108nn62–63, 108n65, 108n67, 108n72, 110n104, 113, 115, 118, 119, 120, 129, 134n3, 134n12, 134nn16–17, 135n28, 135n32, 135n34, 135nn38–39, 135n43, 135n47, 136n56, 136n60, 136n62, 136n74, 136n78, 137n84, 137n87, 137n98
Mahfouz, Naguib 86
Manzalaoui, Mahmoud 106n12

Manifest 20, 23, 53, 57, 63–64, 67, 68, 69, 104
Mann, Thomas 20, 22, 33n36
Mansfield, Katherine 28
Marxism 6 7
Maskelyne (A character in the *Quartet*) 19
Melisa (A character in the *Quartet*) 18, 19, 46, 50, 51, 99
Memory 13, 15, 18, 54n23, 56, 59, 88, 94, 95, 96, 114–115, 121; childhood 27; city of 28, 102, 103; collective 66; disturbing 66; elusive 46; homeland 31; pattern 59; repressed 20, 102; screen 20, 23, 45; rubble 119; being sick 115
Menasce, Alexandria family 68, 129, 130
Menuhin, Diana Gould 91
Menuhin, Yehudi 91
Meyer, C. F. 20
Meltzer, Donald 58
Miller, Alice 135n44
Miller, Henry vii, viii, 6, 7, 8, 9, 10, 31, 107n54, 111–112, 119, 122, 126–127; *The Books in My Life* 134n19, 135n41; letters x, 23, 34n44, 59, 79, 80, 81, 83, 87, 90, 91, 92, 100, 106n23, 113, 116, 127, 131, 133; meeting Durrell x, 129, 130; *Sexus* 112, 134n7; *Tropic of Cancer* 5, 112, 127–128, 134n6, 136n75
Mind, the 10, 20, 21, 40, 44, 45, 54n23, 57, 62, 63, 65, 74, 76, 78, 94, 96, 101, 102, 139
Mitchell, Stephen: *Object Relations in Psychoanalytic Theory* 34n58, 106n9
Modern love 5, 13, 50, 68, 70
Moore, Harry T. 134n17
Morcos, Mona 77, 106n14
Moreno, Elie 108n58
Morris, Jan viii, 78, 106n15
Mother-City 74–105; Alexandria as 93–96; author, *the Heraldic Universe* and loneliness 79–87; Durrell, Freud, Fliess and bisexuality 96–100; Durrell, Groddeck, sexuality and death 100–102; the return 102–105; topographic return to Alexandria 76–79
Mott, Francis John 48
Mountolive, David (A character in the *Quartet*) 19, 28, 49, 55n29, 55n40, 57, 65, 119, 121, 122
Mountolive (Third volume of the *Quartet*) x, 12n27, 28, 32n4, 34n41, 35n66, 35n81, 42, 49, 55n29, 73n25, 73n31, 73n33, 73n35, 102, 135n46, 136n54, 136n58
Mourning 74, 91, 123
Muslim 19, 49, 67, 68, 86, 88, 137n86
Myers, Nancy Isabel (wife) 6, 78
Nabokov, Vladimir 9, 26
Nachträglich 27
Nägele, Rainer 33n29
Naipaul, W. S. 28
Nambiar, Ravindran: *Indian Metaphysics in Lawrence Durrell's Novels* viii
Narrator: critical commentator 52–53; wounded hero 50–52
Narrative voices 7, 13, 37–40, 45, 47–50, 51, 52, 53, 55n29, 57, 60, 61, 83, 99, 104, 123, 140; anonymous 62; choir 47, 66; dominant 48, 87; dreamy, innocent 62; main 17, 46, 49, 78, multiple 32n2, 37, 39, 46, 50, 139; prefatory notes 40–44; *see also* Narrator
Narouz (character in the *Quartet*) 95
Nazi 32n11, 88
Nessim (character in the *Quartet*) 18–19, 30, 48, 49, 51, 53, 66, 67, 68, 69–70, 86, 97, 102, 112, 120
Nietzsche, Friedrich 83, 93–94, 107n37, 107n40, 107n42, 108n78; *On the Genealogy of Morality* 83–84, 107n36, 107n39
Nightingale, Florence 116
Nin, Anaïs vii, viii, 4, 6, 11n13, 75, 105n5, 111, 113, 129, 130, 134n2, 134n19, 137n81, 137n83
Nobel Prize 2
Novel, the 2, 5, 10, 14, 17, 21, 22, 24, 30, 33n20, 36, 48, 49, 50, 60, 61, 77, 85, 89, 112, 123, 124, 129
Nunquam viii, xi, 10, 36

Object, the actual 77, 106n11; internal 76–77, 86, 95; relations 25
Objective 16, 44, 58, 103; data 14; dimension 49; facts 71; light 62; truth 43
Object Relations, school of 34n58, 106n9
Oedipal: complex 96; sexuality 105; world 104, 105
Ogden, Benjamin H.: "The Analyst's Ear and the Critic's Ear" 33n32
Ogden, Thomas 21, 59; "The Analyst's Ear and the Critic's Ear" 33n32; *The Hands of Gravity and Chance* 33n32; *The Parts Left Out* 33n32
Old Tarquin (character in *The Black Book*) 125
Ondaatje, Michael 9
Orient/Oriental 5, 85, 86, 89, 99
Orwell, George 6, 31, 35n83
Other, The 27, 77, 104, 106n11; Oriental 85

Palestine 2, 19, 49, 52, 53, 68–69, 88, 89, 130
Panic Spring x, 136n63

Paris viii, 127, 128; 1937 x, 6, 81, 130; 1938: publication of *The Black Book* x, 35n82
Parker, Kim 30
Pedaya, Haviva 29, 35n72, 35n74, 74, 105n3
Pessoa, Fernando 30
Perlès, Alfred 6, 12n23
Perspective 5, 9, 46, 49, 64, 70, 82, 83, 106n12; Alexandria 75–76, 79, 140; contemporary 41; different 38, 63, 125; interpretive 39; mother-city 140; narrative 13, 123; psychoanalytic 95; Sappho's relationship with mother 116, 133; wider 47; writers 30
Phantasies 20, 24
Pine, Richard 8, 10, 40; *Lawrence Durrell* 11n11, 12n32, 12n45, 54n25, 72n17, 113, 117, 134n11, 134n14, 135n37, 136n73; *Minor Mythologies as Popular Literature* 136n63
Placebo, The viii, 10
Plot 18–19; three layers 46–47
Plutarch 51, 55n43
Poetic influence 3
Poetic space 67, 76, 95, 98, 139, 140
Political 6–8
Porter, Roger 9, 108n61
Pombal (character in the *Quartet*) 18
Pontalis, Jean-Bertrand: *The Language of Psychoanalysis* 54n7
Population: Alexandria 89; Egyptian 38, 86; European refugee 89; local 86, 88, 90, 93; middle class Anglo-Indians 121; Muslim 86; surrounding 114
Post-Structuralism 25
Preconscious 45, 46, 46
Prefatory notes 37, 38–39, 47, 70, 71, 78, 139; narrative voice 40–44
Primal: experience 63, 76, 77; Jewish myth 29; part of the self 32n8; place of belonging 84; satisfaction 26; words 58; wound 134n11
Primeval: city 94; Eden 102, 139; existential conditions 29; experience 5, 18, 65, 74, 75, 95, 105, 120; haven 91; home 88; homeland 10, 22, 117; maternal place 95; motherland 130; place 65, 84; sense of self 61; space 67; state 80, 133; text 48
Primary 31, 77
Prospero's Cell x
Psychoanalysis: interpretation and *The Alexandria Quartet* 22–26; literature 19–22
Psyche 15, 45, 86, 102
Psychic pain 18, 90
Psychotherapy 34n56, 94
Projection 20, 57, 85, 86
Projective identification 85
Protagonist 3, 7, 13, 14, 17, 18, 21, 22, 25, 26, 30, 32n2, 33n21, 36, 38, 39, 42, 43, 45, 46, 47, 52, 53, 57, 66, 69, 70, 71, 75, 78, 79, 80, 95, 96, 98, 101, 105, 118, 124, 134n4, 136n64, 139; central 76; female 49, 99, 104; main 5, 55n29, 67; sexually wounded 50
Proust, Marcel 4, 30, 43, 90
Pursewarden (character in the *Quartet*) 7, 14, 19, 24, 25, 27, 32n8, 38, 39, 40, 48, 49, 52, 53, 55n40, 83
Pynchon, Thomas 9

Quinodoz, Jean-Michel: *Reading Freud* 54n7

Raison d'être 43, 49, 52, 79
Rank, Otto 3, 23, 48, 114–115, 135n27; *Art and Artist* viii
Ray, Man 6
Read, Herbert
Reader, the 4, 5, 8, 10, 11n10, 16, 21, 24, 31, 38, 39, 40, 41, 42, 43–44, 45, 47, 50–51, 59, 63, 64, 66, 67, 68, 71, 72n7, 85, 103, 111
Reading 3, 4, 5–6, 7, 8, 9, 10, 10n1, 11nn10–11, 14, 16, 18, 20, 21, 22, 23, 24, 25, 33, 37, 38, 39, 40, 41, 43, 44, 46, 47, 48, 50, 53, 54n7, 57, 58, 60, 63, 64, 65, 66, 72n7, 72n18, 76, 97, 100, 106n23, 107n44, 109n93, 111, 116, 117, 132, 135n41, 138
Reflective process 16, 24, 25, 28, 36, 37, 39, 40, 41, 50, 53, 57, 59, 65, 71, 75, 76, 133, 138, 139, 140
Refugee 86, 88, 89, 90, 123
Repression 45, 104
Return, the 102–105
Return of the repressed 94, 102, 139
Return, the topographic 76–79
Reverberation 76, 122
Rhodes 26, 92, 93
Richard III 123–124
Ridler, Anne 90
Rilke, Rainer Maria 15, 20
Rimbaud, Arthur 103, 110n116
Robson, Barbara 9, 12n49, 133, 137n91
Roessel, David 10haag
Roth, Merav: *Reading the Reader* 11n10
Rolland, Romain 14
Roman Empire, The (Rome) 51, 110n116
Rushdie, Salman: *Imaginary Homelands* 34n50

Sagi, Avi 15, 32n9
Sandler, Joseph 34n55

Schiller, Friedrich 20
Schleiermacher, Friedrich 16, 33n14
Schnitzler, Arthur 20
Screen memory 23, 45
Second World War 5, 26, 27, 39, 47, 49, 75, 88, 103, 128
Secret wound 3, 18, 61, 111–134, 139; childhood *Kim* years 113–115; *see also* Durrell, Louisa
Seidel, Michael 29, 35n75
Shakespeare, Hamnet 18
Shakespeare, John 18
Shakespeare, William 18, 20, 123; *Hamlet* 17–18; *Richard III* 123–124
Simpson, John 35n70
Self 22, 27, 32n8, 45, 52, 63, 82, 96, 101, 115, 119; -absorbed 130; –analysis viii; -assessment viii; -centred 38; cohesion 53; complex 47; -debasing 124; -defence 109n85; -disclosure 112; -discovery 30, 79, 140; -disintegration 124; -doubt 50; duplicate 2; -expression 53, 81, 140; fragmented entity 31; free rein 53; -fulfilment 2, 5, 7, 67, 79, 138, 140; -hatred 119; -knowledge 140; lost 139; mental processes 59; nature 48; non-uniform 48; part 21, 32n8, 76; -portrait 17; respect 92; sense 2, 59, 60, 61, 85; split 48; -study 83
Sex 10, 25, 92, 101, 122; contact 64; debauchery 93; drives 52, 64, 73n27; ecstasy 98; experiences 75, 89, 91, 98, 105, 124, 126; forbidden desires 65, 86; horizons 89; incest 104, 108n63, 132; perverse 65, 86, 103, 104, 140; responses 90; wishes 103
Sexuality 5, 7, 10, 25, 26, 28, 36, 45, 53, 75, 94, 97, 98–104, 109n93, 112, 115, 119, 140; bisexuality 97, 98, 100–101, 109n93; centrality 97; childhood 15, 104; dreams 57; female 100; feminine 70; homosexuality 109n93; illicit 55n40; infantile 23; Oedipal 105; oppression 110n119; Oriental 99; phantasies 20, 65; psychosexual development 15; raw 13; repressed 16; salvation 98; wild 85; wounded 50, 97, 98, 125
Shamir, Kibbutz 2
Sickness 50, 75, 100, 101, 102, 115; *see also* Disease; Illness
Silence 24, 92, 94
Sligh, Charles L. 8, 12n44
Slips of the tongue 23, 45
Solitude 2, 37, 51, 80, 81, 82, 83, 84, 85, 118, 128, 138, 140; pain 117
Sommières 9
South of France 9, 27, 42, 76, 79, 88, 113, 125, 129, 130, 132
Spence, Donald 22, 33n37, 71, 73n38
Spero, Moshe Halevi 59, 72n11, 72n15
Spirit of Place 106n16, 108n66, 108n71, 135n23, 136n68, 136n77, 137n99
Steiner, George 8, 12n36, 19, 22, 33n25, 34n42, 74, 105n1
Storr, Anthony 73n27, 82, 107n32
Structure 44–46
Subject 30, 31, 38, 71, 72n8, 78, 87, 120
Subjective 16, 43, 60, 62; content 99; experience 34n56, 38, 47, 68, 75, 117; identity 32; object 77; sense of time 38; time 38, 139
Sublimation 29, 53, 57, 75
Superego 25, 32n8, 37, 45, 48, 52, 53
Surrealist/Surrealism vii, 6, 7, 80
Swift, Jonathan 64, 65
Symptoms 17, 29, 45, 47, 53, 94

Testimony 3, 17, 29, 30, 37, 40, 41, 47, 50, 83, 132
Thompson, Edward 35n73
Tibet 117
Time, chronological 44, 80
Time, subjective 38, 139
Theory of relativity 38, 39, 43, 44, 139
Topography 37, 45, 46, 61, 101, 139
Topographical models of the mind 10
Trauma 29, 42, 56, 60, 63, 65, 84, 89, 94, 115
Travel 3, 9, 64, 75, 87, 93, 118, 123, 129
Truth i, 3, 13, 23, 25, 36, 46, 52–53, 57, 62, 63, 70, 76, 84, 96, 101, 103, 105, 109n85, 111–112; aspiration 70–71; contradictory 71; historical 22, 67, 70, 71; narrative 22, 58, 71; objective 43; paradoxical 71; relativity 44, 130; reliability 61; transcendental 140
Tunc vii, viii, xi, 10, 32n13, 36
Turner, Victor 35n68, 98, 109n96

Unconscious vii, 2, 14, 15, 16, 17, 18, 20, 21, 22, 24, 26, 37, 39, 41, 44, 45, 47, 48, 50, 53, 57, 58, 59, 60, 65, 66, 72n7, 75, 76, 77, 78, 83, 85, 87, 94, 96, 103, 110n113, 139, 140
Das unheimliche (The Uncanny) 1, 2, 14, 22, 26, 27, 30, 32n8, 42, 45, 46, 56, 58,

65, 67, 69, 71, 90, 93, 94, 95, 103, 114, 120, 123, 124, 134, 138, 139
Unterecker, John 113, 135n20

Vassanji, M. G. 9
Villa Seurat 12n24, 127
Vincendon, Claude-Marie/Claude (Third Wife) 43; death 9, 81, 130, 131, 132, 133

Walsh, W. H. 70, 73n37
Weigel, John A. 38, 54n13, 113, 135n21, 135n36
Whitman, Aldan 54n5
Wickes, George 12n28
Weltanschauung 50, 80
Williams, Gwyn 108n58
Wish 14, 26, 45, 52, 54n10, 56, 60, 64, 65, 67, 83, 95, 98, 104, 105, 118, 120, 122, 126, 127
Woman, the 52, 69, 70, 73n34, 91, 99, 100, 101, 102
Workpoints 40, 43, 44, 47, 55n29, 71, 139
Winnicott, D. W. 106n11

Young, Kenneth 54n11

Zeus 109n85
Zionist Movement 68
Zweig, Stefen 20
Zahaln, Anne 107n45
Ziffer, Benny 10n1